2004

THE ESSENTIAL
C-SECTION GUIDE

THE ESSENTIAL C-SECTION GUIDE

Pain Control, Healing at Home,

Getting Your Body Back

— AND EVERYTHING ELSE

You Need to Know About

a Cesarean Birth

Maureen Connolly AND *Dana Sullivan*

Broadway Books
New York

BROADWAY

Broadway Books titles may be purchased for business or promotional use or for special sales. For information, please write to: Special Markets Department, Random House, Inc., 1745 Broadway, New York, NY 10019.

PRINTED IN THE UNITED STATES OF AMERICA

BROADWAY BOOKS and its logo, a letter B bisected on the diagonal, are trademarks of Random House, Inc.

Visit our website at www.broadwaybooks.com

First edition published 2004.

Book design by Fearn Cutler deVicq
Illustrated by Jackie Aher

Library of Congress Cataloging-in-Publication Data

Connolly, Maureen.
The Essential C-Section Guide: Pain Control, Healing at Home, Getting Your Body Back and Everything Else You Need to Know About a Cesarean Birth by Maureen Connolly and Dana Sullivan.—1st ed.
    p.   cm.
Includes bibliographical references and index.
ISBN 0-7679-1607-7
1. Cesarean section—Popular works.   2. Mothers—Health and hygiene—Popular works.
3. Self-care, Health.   I. Sullivan, Dana.   II. Title.
RG761.C66 2004
618.8'6—dc22   2003063582

1   3   5   7   9   10   8   6   4   2

Contents

Acknowledgments

We would not have been able to write this book without generous help from the professionals who made sure that, medically speaking, our i's were dotted and our t's crossed: Katherine E. Economy, MD, M.P.H., a maternal-fetal specialist and academic instructor at Harvard Medical School and Brigham and Women's Hospital in Boston. William R. Camann, MD, director of obstetric anesthesia at Brigham and Women's Hospital and professor of anesthesia at Harvard Medical School; Sharon Phelan, MD, FACOG, professor of obstetrics and gynecology at the University of New Mexico Health Science Center in Albuquerque; Luis Sanchez-Ramos, MD, professor of perinatal medicine in the department of obstetrics and gynecology at the University of Florida in Jacksonville; Zane A. Brown, MD, professor of perinatal medicine in the department of obstetrics and gynecology at the University of Washington in Seattle; Alice Domar, PhD, director of the Mind/Body Center for Women's Health at Boston IVF; Cheston Berlin, MD, professor of pediatrics and pharmacy, at the Pennsylvania State University College of Medicine in Hershey; Michael Milano, MD, an obstetrician gynecologist in private practice in Verona, N.J.; James Lemons, MD, director of the neonatology section at the James Whitcomb Riley Hospital for Children and professor of pediatrics at the Indiana University School of

Medicine in Indianapolis; Andy Spooner, MD, director of the department of pediatrics at University of Tennessee Health Sciences Center College of Medicine in Memphis; Robert Lorenz, MD, a spokesperson for the American College of Obstetricians and Gynecologists. Alice Kirkman and Gregory Phillips of ACOG made sure we spoke with the right people.

Our thanks to the Association of Women's Health, Obstetric and Neonatal Nurses (AWHONN) for arranging interviews with nurses who know better than anyone what a c-section patient goes through: Sharyn Grzeszczak, RN, CEN, obstetric clinical coordinator, St. Barnabas Medical Center, Livingston, N.J.; Renee Jones, RNC, MSN, critical care obstetrics and recovery, Presbyterian Hospital of Dallas; Molly Kealy, RN, BSN, labor and delivery, Anne Arundel Medical Center in Annapolis.

Our gratitude to Alexandra Spadola, MD, an obstetrics resident at Columbia-Presbyterian's Sloane Hospital for Women and Children, who let us sit with her one morning and pick her brain about her experiences delivering babies. Susan E.C. Sorensen, MD, a pediatrician in Reno, answered many questions about how babies fare following a Cesarean birth. Thank you.

To the professionals who shared their knowledge about how a c-section surgery can affect women emotionally: Deborah Issokson, PsyD, a licensed psychologist and director of Counseling for Reproductive Health and Healing, a private practice based in Watertown, Mass.; Diana Lynn Barnes, PsyD, a marriage and family therapist and president of Postpartum Support International, a nonprofit organization based in Woodland Hills, Calif.; Shellie Fidell, MSW, LCSW, a counselor with the Women's Healthcare Partnership in St. Louis; David Diamond, PhD, director of The Center for Reproductive Psychology, a nonprofit organization affiliated with Alliant International University-California School of Professional Psychology in San

Diego; Tamara Gibson, a doctoral student at Alliant International University-California School of Professional Psychology in San Diego. Your insights were invaluable.

We know that the information from Katy Lebbing of La Leche League International; Linda Donovan, RN, a board-certified lactation consultant; and Dottie James, PhD, RN, coordinator of the perinatal graduate nursing specialty at Saint Louis University School of Nursing, will give many readers the confidence they need to breast-feed. Lynn A. Millar, PT, PhD, a professor of physical therapy at Andrews University in Berrien Springs, Mich.; Elizabeth Joy, MD, an associate professor in the department of family and preventative medicine at the University of Utah–Salt Lake City; and Michelle Mottola, PhD, of the University of Western Ontario in Canada, offered advice on getting back into shape. Heidi Reichenberger, MS, RD, weighed in with some important information about nutrition. Debi Pillarella, MEd, created a postCesarean exercise program that is more than we could have wished for (and wish we'd had ourselves after our own deliveries). Information about sex after a Cesarean, which came from Lisa Douglass, PhD, will help many readers rediscover intimacy after pregnancy and childbirth. Pam Warren, RN, a nurse at St. Mary's Hospital in Reno, shared advice on healing at home. Thank you all. Our agent Kristen Auclair was very patient in helping two novices navigate the treacherous waters that are book publishing. Rebecca Geiger made sure that we had our facts straight and that our research was on the money. Tricia Medved, our editor at Broadway Books, believed in this book right from the start. Thank you. Without the moms who shared their experiences with us and offered their own tried-and-true advice, we wouldn't have such a well-rounded resource. We're so grateful that you willingly shared your stories.

—*Dana and Maureen*

Maureen Connolly had the idea for this book, and I am honored that she thinks enough of me to have had me collaborate with her. I can't imagine a better accomplice and only regret that we live so far apart. Suzanne Schlosberg was instrumental in helping us shape a germ of an idea into a bona fide proposal—thank you, thank you. I'm grateful to my sister-in-law, Stephanie Kilroy, and my friend, Traci B. Pitts, PhD, whose careful reading of drafts of early chapters was very helpful. I am blessed to have the most wonderful friends a person could ask for. You know who you are—thank you. I cherish my parents, Betty and Roger, who are so proud that you'd think I'd written the Great American Novel. My husband, Robert Kilroy, was, as always, my biggest cheerleader and gave me the space and support I needed to get this project done. To him and to our children, Liam and Julia, plus our newest addition, Carina: my heart is full of you.

—D.S.

I may have had the idea for this project, but my coauthor Dana Sullivan was instrumental in getting us started and seeing us through to a more impressive end than I could ever have achieved on my own. Thanks to my two wonderful sisters, and my parents, whose love never wavers, and who nearly four decades later continue to teach me that all things are possible. To Alicia, my friend and confidant, for sharing our enthusiasm for this book and agreeing to get the word out about it! John Connolly, thank you for the endless hours of tech support, coffee refills, and pep talks—but most important, for believing more than anyone that I could succeed at this. And last, but most certainly not least, my two little guys Jack and Sean—if it weren't for your adorable, big, Irish heads, I would never have been sitting here writing this.

—M.C.

Foreword

During the ten years that I have been practicing medicine I have witnessed many changes in obstetrics. We have learned much over the last decade about the safety of Cesarean delivery. And improvements in surgical techniques, antibiotics, anesthesia, and postpartum care have minimized risks of infection, hemorrhage, and post-operative complications. In some instances, a c-section may be a safer option for both mother and baby than a vaginal birth.

As the number of Cesarean deliveries continues to increase, we as providers face many new challenges. Despite the fact that more than one in four women delivers by Cesarean, there is still a culture of fear and failure surrounding this mode of delivery. So one of our goals as physicians caring for pregnant women is to educate them not only about pregnancy and vaginal birth, but also about the very real possibility of delivering by Cesarean and what that entails.

It's important for all pregnant women to understand that having a "normal" pregnancy and a "normal" birth experience doesn't necessarily mean a vaginal delivery. Once a woman goes into labor things can change very quickly: a surgical delivery can become necessary in a matter of minutes. In other cases, a c-section is the end result of many hours of labor.

Because the focus of many childbirth education programs is on vaginal birth, I find that when I recommend to my patients that they deliver by Cesarean, they—understandably—have lots of questions. And they are often nervous about the prospect. Even with reassurances that modern advances have made Cesarean delivery incredibly safe, the thought of having a surgical birth still makes most women uncomfortable. (Since I specialize in high-risk pregnancies, the percentage of my patients who are candidates for c-sections is even higher than average.) As a maternal-fetal specialist, my job is to care for women during a time when they already feel like they don't have much control over what is happening to their bodies. When the possibility of a Cesarean birth first arises, I am careful to answer my patients' questions, educate them about what's involved in a surgical birth, and of course, reassure them that they and their baby will be safe. Thanks to this book, my job will be a little bit easier from now on. Pregnant women facing a Cesarean delivery, and those who have recently experienced a surgical birth, will find *The Essential C-Section Guide* an invaluable resource.

In these pages, you'll find frank, thoroughly researched, and comforting answers to common questions about a c-section birth. From "How much will it hurt?" to "What does this c-section mean for future pregnancies?" to "When can I start exercising again?" Maureen Connolly and Dana Sullivan have addressed virtually every issue that pertains to this topic.

Recently there has been a fair amount of controversy surrounding the relatively high rate of c-sections performed in the United States. Even though the authors had their own children by Cesarean, they do not "endorse" this as the preferred method of childbirth. In fact, they are careful to include discussions about the challenges and risks associated with the surgery and what's involved with the recovery and its impact on future pregnancies.

When it comes to birth by Cesarean, there is opinion and there is fact. In these pages readers will find little of the former and plenty of the latter. And they will also find wisdom, support, and practical advice. If all of my patients read this book before their c-sections, or in the days, weeks, even months afterward, I am certain they would feel more comfortable about the path that pregnancy has taken them on, and they would be able to enjoy the birth experience regardless of the mode of delivery.

—*Katherine E. Economy, MD, M.P.H., maternal-fetal specialist and academic instructor at Harvard Medical School and Brigham and Women's Hospital in Boston*

Introduction

I f you picked up this book, you are likely to fall into one of the following four categories:

- You have just had a Cesarean and are wondering what's in store for your physical and/or emotional recovery.
- You recently learned that you're going to deliver your baby via Cesarean and you have a few days, weeks, or months to educate yourself about what's ahead.
- You have had at least one Cesarean birth, are pregnant again, and want to be better prepared for the experience in case you have a repeat.
- You're pregnant and just want to be sure you have your bases covered. With the rates of birth by Cesarean rising in the United States, you want to know what to expect, just in case.

Whichever one best describes you, *this book will help.*

We wrote this book because we wanted to provide women with the information that we wish we'd had when we delivered our babies by Cesarean—five of them between us—just a few years ago. If a Cesarean birth is in your future, you undoubtedly have questions: *How much pain should I be prepared for? Are babies delivered by c-section at higher risk for health problems? Will*

I be able to breast-feed? Will a Cesarean surgery affect my sex life? Afterward you may wonder: *How can I relieve this horrible gas pain? When can I start exercising? Will my stomach ever be flat again? Why do I feel like a failure?* We have the answers.

We spoke with dozens of medical experts around the country and consulted medical journals and textbooks so that we could walk you step-by-step through the surgery. We researched such topics as the most common reasons Cesareans are performed, what women need to know if they plan to breast-feed, and what is critical for healing following a surgical delivery. We also interviewed moms who had Cesarean births and asked them to share their experiences. We include a comprehensive exercise program that will help you get fit—a challenge for any new mom, but especially for those who've had abdominal surgery.

Looking back on our own Cesarean experiences, we both realize now how utterly unprepared we were for them. We'd taken childbirth education classes and read a dozen pregnancy books between us, but neither of us thought we'd be the "one in four." Most of the pregnancy books we read, even our favorites, include just a few pages about Cesarean birth and recovery from it. What's more, the bulk of the information about c-sections that does exist focuses on how to avoid them. The reality is that each year more than one million women in the United States undergo this procedure. We feel strongly that more attention needs to be given to Cesarean education. Cesarean surgery has saved the lives of countless women and babies in the last century. And childbirth is a miracle no matter how the baby is brought into the world.

The purpose of this book is not to debate whether Cesarean deliveries occur too often in this country. We'll leave that argument to the physicians, midwives, doulas, insurance company representatives, and attorneys. Our ultimate goal is simply to help women be better prepared for a Cesarean birth, and to help with their physical and emotional recovery.

A few notes: you will discover throughout the book that we usually refer to the people who deliver babies as physicians or obstetricians. While we acknowledge that nurses and midwives play a primary role in both prenatal care and childbirth, only physicians are licensed to perform Cesarean deliveries in this country. For that reason, we also most often refer to the place where babies are born as hospitals, rather than birthing centers. We do not intend to diminish the role that nonphysician care-givers play in the labor-and-delivery process, nor do we wish to suggest that only physicians are capable of delivering babies, just that in the context of Cesarean surgery, they are the ones responsible.

Regarding the use of pronouns; throughout the book we use "he" when referring to babies and we use "she" when referring to physicians.

We should also point out that physicians do not prefer the terms Cesarean section and c-section. There are many theories about where the term "Cesarean" comes from (more on that later), and one is that it derives from two Latin words, *caedre* and *secare*, which both mean "to cut." Since "section" also means "to cut," the terms Cesarean section and c-section are re-dundant. That said, nearly every woman who delivers a baby via Cesarean refers to it as a "c-section," hence the title of our book.

CHAPTER 1

Why a Cesarean?

"'Don't cut her open, she's not numb!' I heard the anesthesiologist yell to my OB as a team of nurses rushed me down the hall toward an operating room. 'Wait, wait, wait!' was all I could think, so stunned that I couldn't even speak. This wasn't how it was supposed to happen. 'But I'm barely in labor,' I managed to say before the anesthesiologist placed a mask over my face and instructed me to breathe. He counted to three and the lights went out. When I woke up later, it was to the news that my newborn son was on life support."

That was how one of our perfect and perfectly uneventful pregnancies (Dana's) ended. In a matter of minutes, labor shifted from ordinary to potentially disastrous and an emergency Cesarean became necessary.

Even though we had completely different experiences with our first Cesareans—Maureen labored for nine hours, pushing for two and a half of them, before it became clear that her son Jack wasn't going to come out any way but through her belly— there were many similar themes. We each had "normal," healthy pregnancies; we both felt very prepared for labor by the end of our childbirth classes; and neither of us even considered the *possibility* that we would have Cesareans. In the weeks after our

babies' births, when we were home and well on the road to recovery following the surgery, we both felt an overwhelming
sense of failure. "*Why me?*" and "*What did I do wrong?*" were
questions we asked ourselves for months.

Making Sense of the Statistics

With the benefit of hindsight, we know that our Cesarean
deliveries weren't the result of anything we did—or didn't do.
But very few pregnant women (at least those who are not carrying multiples or have certain medical conditions) plan even
for the possibility that they will give birth via c-section. More of
us should; the odds that a baby born in the United States will
be delivered via Cesarean are more than one in four, 26.1 percent to be exact; 18 percent of the Cesareans performed in 2002
were primary, that is, performed on women who had not had a
previous Cesarean delivery.

During the past few years, there has been a lot of controversy surrounding these statistics. A number of healthcare
providers, including some OB/GYNs, believe that the Cesarean
birth rate in the United States is too high and, in many cases,
that surgical deliveries are unnecessary. "We have turned childbirth into a medical procedure," is a frequent refrain. While we
certainly don't believe that a Cesarean is the ideal way to give
birth—and we would never encourage anyone to request a
c-section for the sake of convenience—neither should women
who have one feel that their birth experience is anything but extraordinary. Childbirth by Cesarean is still childbirth. It's also
worth noting one fact that is rarely brought up by the media:
medical advances during the last several decades have made
c-section surgery much safer, so today many physicians will opt
for a Cesarean birth well before the situation becomes desper-
ate.

The fact that the technique now used in about 90 percent of all c-sections—called a "low transverse" incision—has fewer complications than the vertical incision that was used for many years is one reason. This refined surgical technique has made it possible for women to attempt a vaginal birth after Cesarean (called a VBAC) in subsequent pregnancies. This makes some physicians less reluctant to perform a Cesarean on a first-time mom. Another reason is developments in anesthesia. Namely, that a regional anesthetic can be used 90 percent of the time, rather than a general, which lowers the risk of complication and death from anesthesia. Now there also are a variety of antibiotics that protect against postoperative infection, which was a substantial risk historically associated with Cesarean deliveries. Finally, the number of women who are delivering babies in their thirties and forties has increased dramatically. Women between the ages of thirty and fifty-four have a 35 percent chance of delivery by Cesarean; women under twenty-nine face a 22 percent chance. (In part, that's because older women face a host of age-related risk factors, including a higher likelihood of experiencing preterm labor, which necessitate a Cesarean delivery to preserve the health of the baby.) Each of these factors has contributed to the increase in Cesarean deliveries.

During the course of our research for this book, we heard two telling comments from physicians. The first was, "When something goes wrong during labor, it generally doesn't go just a little bit wrong. Things can go from bad to tragic in a matter of minutes." The second was, "The few inches that a baby travels during childbirth is the most dangerous distance he'll travel during his whole life." With those two thoughts in mind, and before we veer into melodrama, let us state that we are grateful that we had emergency obstetric delivery options available to us. Until the early 1900s, both babies and mothers were not always expected to survive a Cesarean delivery in this country. In many parts of the world today, women still don't have the procedure available to them—and the cost in human lives is heartbreaking.

The History of the Cesarean

It is generally believed that the term "Cesarean" originated with the surgical birth of Julius Caesar. At the time of his birth, babies were delivered surgically in order to save the life of a baby whose mother was dying or already dead. But it is known that Julius Caesar's mother, Aurelia, was alive at least long enough to hear of her son's invasion of Britain—making it unlikely that his was a surgical birth. A more plausible origin for the term may have to do with Roman law under Caesar, which required that women who were beyond saving during childbirth be cut open in order to preserve the life of the baby. Babies were highly valued because they added numbers to the country's population. Another theory is that the term comes from the Latin words *caedre*, which means "to cut," or *caesones*, a label that was given to babies who were born after their mothers had died.

The first successful Cesarean delivery using Western medical techniques is credited to a female physician named James Miranda Stuart Barry, who was masquerading as a man (women were generally denied admission to medical schools) and serving in the British Army in South Africa. The surgery took place sometime between 1815 and 1821. Dr. Barry's surgical delivery probably wasn't the first successful surgical delivery in the world, however. Europeans traveling in Uganda and Rwanda in the nineteenth century also reported witnessing surgical deliveries. In these deliveries the "healer" would use wine to sedate the patient and pin the incision closed with iron needles instead of Western-style sutures.

In the mid-nineteenth century, a Massachusetts dentist successfully used diethyl ether to anesthetize a patient so he could remove a facial tumor. After that, anesthesia became widely used for many surgical procedures. It took some years before anesthesia was used for Cesareans, however, because women were still expected to "sorrow"—i.e., suffer in pain—as they brought children into the world. In the later nineteenth and early twentieth centuries, advancements in anesthesia and antiseptic formulas made it possible for surgeons to operate slowly and to properly cleanse the abdominal region, which prevented women from dying of infection and shock. By the early twentieth century, the availability of penicillin significantly reduced the number of women who died as a result of infection.

Why a Cesarean Today?

Fast forward to the twenty-first century. We now have tools that can accurately gauge how a pregnancy is progressing at every stage. By monitoring both maternal and fetal health, physicians are able to prepare for or react to situations that make a vaginal birth risky or impossible. There are dozens of scenarios that lead to Cesarean deliveries today—and unlike Roman law, none is aimed at increasing the population! Many situations develop only moments before the physician decides it's time to get the baby out, either because the mother's or the baby's health is jeopardized. In other cases, both the doctor and the expectant mother know early in pregnancy that delivery via c-section is a distinct possibility. The mom-to-be may have a medical condition, such as high blood pressure, heart disease, or diabetes, that makes Cesarean the safest mode of delivery for her. She may be infected with HIV or hepatitis C, or, the baby may have spina bifida or hydrocephalus, which make surgical delivery the safer route for the baby.

On occasion, physicians know at the very first prenatal visit that Cesarean is the most likely way the baby will be delivered: the mother may have fibroids that block the birth canal, or she may have a malformed pelvis due to a birth defect or an improperly healed pelvic injury. Delivering twins by Cesarean used to be routine, but today only about half of twin deliveries are surgical. The rate is higher for triplets and higher order multiples. Typically, multiples have higher rates of Cesarean deliveries than singletons because often they need to be delivered prematurely and are smaller than lone babies, both factors that put them at risk for experiencing life-threatening distress during labor.

While we cannot cover every circumstance that results in a c-section, there are a few major "indications"—to borrow the medical term—for Cesarean delivery:

Previous c-section

A prior Cesarean is the number-one reason for a surgical delivery in the United States, accounting for more than one-third of all procedures (see Table 1, "By the Numbers"). A woman who has had one c-section has better than an 80 percent chance that she'll have another with her future pregnancies.

Even though the percentage of women delivering vaginally following a Cesarean has decreased—to roughly 13 percent in 2002—that 80 percent c-section rate is actually a relative improvement. Until about the mid-1950s, once a woman had had one Cesarean, the chances that subsequent deliveries would also be surgical was close to 100 percent. That's because before the widespread use of the low transverse incision, also known as a "bikini cut," the surgical technique used for Cesarean deliveries was the "classical cut." This type of incision left the woman with a long vertical scar that weakened the uterus, making it more likely to rupture during future pregnancies and deliveries. Today the classical cut is used in certain emergency situations, if the baby is lying sideways, in what's called the transverse position or if the baby is very premature or breech.

Dystocia, aka, a difficult labor

We know, there's no such thing as an easy labor! However, *dystocia* (dis-tow-sha) is something more than run-of-the-mill labor discomfort. Dystocia is the second most common reason cited for Cesarean delivery. The term describes a labor that has failed to progress or has become otherwise "dysfunctional," making the birth attendants feel that the baby's or the mother's safety—or both—is in danger. Reasons for a difficult labor may include a mother with a narrow pelvis, making it difficult for her to deliver a large baby (called "cephalopelvic disproportion"). It may be that the contractions aren't strong enough either to dilate the cervix fully, or to push the baby all the way through the birth canal, or it might be a combination of any of these factors.

A change of plans

"A week before my official due date, my obstetrician delivered the news that my daughter would probably need to be delivered via Cesarean. A sonogram showed that the baby had an unusually large head and chest; the doctor estimated her weight at nine pounds, four ounces. I'm a petite woman and have a narrow pelvis, but I was distraught when he recommended the Cesarean. When I saw her head afterward, even though I was disappointed I didn't have a vaginal birth, I was also relieved. At first I felt vulnerable for letting my doctor make this decision, but I am also thankful that I could trust him. In the end I know we did the right thing. And his estimate was right on: Emma came into the world weighing exactly nine pounds, four ounces."

—Tracey, mother of one, a Cesarean in 1998

Some women who wind up having Cesareans due to dystocia are strong and healthy and experience labor that progresses without a hitch until the cervix dilates all the way to ten centimeters. But if the baby hasn't descended into the birth canal, either because he is too large or mom's pelvis is too small, or his head is positioned in a vulnerable way, the obstetrician or midwife has a difficult decision to make. At this point the physician can recommend non-medical intervention, such as an hour of rest or a change of position. A midwife or nurse may give you a massage, or a bath (if your water hasn't broken). The labor and delivery attendants may decide to try to help both mom and Mother Nature along by administering Pitocin, a drug that strengthens contractions. Or the healthcare provider may decide to rupture the amniotic sac.

All these options fall into a category called "active management of labor," and may help the birthing process progress. But at a certain point, if labor doesn't respond to such interventions, a Cesarean is usually necessary. When labor stalls for more than about an hour—the official term is "arrest of labor"—it indicates that one of the body's protective mechanisms has kicked in. The uterus will basically stop contracting, which stalls labor and leaves the baby in a precarious place. In this situation, a surgical delivery may be called for in order to prevent a potentially catastrophic outcome.

Fetal heart rate abnormality, also called fetal distress

Most hospitals and even some birthing centers rely on fetal heart rate monitoring to measure a baby's status. The monitor measures the heart rate both during contractions—from the beginning to the end of one—and from one stage of labor to the next. If the heart-rate pattern looks abnormal, it may mean the umbilical cord is being squeezed, suggesting that the baby is being deprived of oxygen. It may also mean the baby isn't positioned for a smooth journey through the birth canal, that there is "uteroplacental insufficiency" (meaning there isn't enough exchange of oxygen between the uterus and the placenta), or that the placenta has abrupted (see below for details).

A normal fetal heart rate is approximately 120 to 160 beats per minute. If the heart-rate decelerates, that is, drops below that level, and doesn't recover quickly when the contraction ends, many physicians will not "wait and see" if baby is going to tolerate more labor, but rather will opt for a Cesarean after about thirty minutes (or less) of repeated decelerations. Likewise, if the heart rate is unusually rapid, it may mean that the baby is having to work too hard to get enough oxygen and that a Cesarean possibly is in order.

The use of fetal heart-rate monitoring as the determining factor in performing a c-section is very controversial and the decision is still subjective. One monitoring option, called a fetal oximetry sensor, involves placing a sensor on the baby's cheek while he's in the birth canal. The sensor measures the oxygen content of the blood through the skin and the physician can determine from it whether the baby is being deprived of oxygen. She can also scrape the baby's scalp to obtain a blood sample. Then the blood is analyzed quickly and if the pH levels in the blood suggest that the baby isn't getting enough oxygen, a Cesarean is likely. Before performing the Cesarean, some doctors will also try additional tests that measure how the baby is doing. For instance, they may try "acoustic stimulation," during which loud noise is used to try to awaken the baby—and reassure the physician that the baby isn't in distress.

Any woman whose c-section delivery was the result of fetal heart-rate abnormality or fetal distress will report that as soon as the labor-and-delivery nurses, midwife, and/or physician no-ticed a "nonreassuring" heart-rate during fetal monitoring, there was a palpable shift in their demeanor. When labor is pro-gressing normally, the nurses are generally calm and reassuring to the laboring mother. But as soon as it's clear that baby is dis-tressed, their tones become clipped, and they start moving around the room with a sense of urgency. And even though mom-to-be is likely doing her best to breathe and to manage her pain, she is acutely aware that something, well, bad may be happening.

That said, doctors freely admit that a diagnosis of fetal dis-tress—or whichever term they favor—is imprecise, and that the decision to perform a c-section based on this diagnosis is sub-jective. "Ask ten OBs at what point they decide that the nonre-assuring heart-rate warrants surgical delivery and you'll get ten different answers," one physician told us. Interestingly, one study found that Cesareans performed due to fetal distress peaked between 9 p.m. and 3 a.m., suggesting that perhaps physicians are less tolerant of fetal heart-rate abnormalities during these late-night hours.

Roughly 10 percent of Cesarean deliveries are the result of fetal heart-rate abnormality. It's important to realize that it's perfectly normal for a baby to display some fluctuations in his heart rate: the birthing process is no picnic for him either. The challenge for the healthcare providers is determining which stresses are reasonable and which potentially could be harmful to the baby.

Malpresentation

To prepare for the journey down the birth canal, most ba-bies turn themselves into the head down position around the thirty-seventh week of pregnancy. Babies who don't turn, however, are generally in one of three positions: *breech*—meaning baby's buttocks remain down or one or both of his legs are "presenting" first; *brow*—meaning the forehead is presenting; or *transverse*—meaning the baby is lying horizontally or at an angle in the uterus. Any of these malpresentations can cause labor to stall.

The main reason that breech babies are often delivered surgically is that if baby descends buttocks or legs first, his head might become stuck in the birth canal after his lower half is out. Since part of the umbilical cord, which contains the baby's oxygen supply, may still remain in the birth canal, there is a risk that the cord will be compressed and the baby, deprived of oxygen, may possibly suffer permanent brain damage or suffocate. A recent study of breech births in twenty-six countries found that babies born vaginally from the frank breech position were three times more likely to suffer serious injury or death than the frank breech babies who were delivered by planned Cesarean. For that reason alone, many physicians won't allow a woman to attempt a vaginal birth if the baby is breech when labor begins.

A more unusual malpresentation is called *brow*. Pretend that you are looking at the stars overhead and bend your head back as far as you can. Now imagine that your whole body is crammed inside a very narrow passageway and your head is utterly stuck in this position. This is what the brow position is like for a baby. When a baby's head is flexed like this, he is in serious jeopardy. As soon as it's evident that the baby is presenting this way, the attending physician will perform a Cesarean.

Finally, if the baby is transverse, or even lying at a 45-degree angle, there is little chance he will come out any way but via Cesarean. Everyone has heard at least one mom say that when she gave birth, she felt like she had pushed a watermelon out of her vagina. Well, to push a transverse baby out would be more like trying to push a La-Z-Boy recliner through an opening that's *just* big enough for a watermelon. It isn't going to happen.

. . . .

A Cesarean after three vaginal births?

"I found out at almost thirty-eight weeks that my baby is feet first and that my doctor thinks versions [when a doctor tries manually to turn the baby to a head-down position] are dangerous and won't do them. He just told me that if the baby doesn't turn to the head-down position by thirty-nine weeks, he will schedule a Cesarean. The danger is that if my water breaks the baby's cord could prolapse, which would be very dangerous for the baby. If that happens, I would have an emergency Cesarean. I've already had three vaginal births; I don't want my fourth and last pregnancy to end with surgery. But since my water has broken with two of my three previous pregnancies, I'm also worried about the baby. I don't want to have abdominal surgery, I don't want a scar. I already know what to expect from a vaginal birth and the recovery, so this is uncharted territory and I have that fear of the unknown. I'm trying to balance my belief that nature will take its course, and that this baby will do what it's supposed to do, with my understanding that both babies and mothers can die in my situation. I am grateful that I have the option to protect my health and my baby's health."

—JulieAnna, mother of three, and a fourth on the way

. . . .

Placental Problems: Placenta Previa, Placenta Accreta, and Placental Abruption

Normally, the placenta forms near the top of the uterus or on the sides. But in *placenta previa*, the placenta implants on the uterine wall either partially (*partial* previa) or entirely (*complete* previa) over the cervix. This not only potentially blocks the baby's exit, but it also makes the uterus susceptible to bleeding.

Once the cervix begins to dilate, the placenta pulls away from the uterine wall, causing bleeding. In fact, placenta previa is usually diagnosed toward the end of pregnancy when painless bleeding occurs, but it can also be noticed in the second trimester during ultrasound. *Placenta previa* is dangerous because it sometimes leads to life-threatening hemorrhage in the mother, either during labor or postpartum. It also increases the risk of *placenta accreta*, a situation in which the placenta has actually burrowed into uterine muscle rather than simply attached itself to the uterine lining. *Placenta accreta* can lead to life-threatening bleeding, or result in the need for an emergency hysterectomy.

Another placental problem, *abruptio placenta* (or placental abruption), means that the placenta has separated, either partially or totally, from the uterine wall, causing bleeding. Placental abruption can happen either late in pregnancy or during labor. In some cases the separation is considered mild; the bleeding is light and bed rest is often the only treatment. If the separation is moderate, the mother can lose enough blood that she requires a transfusion; if she is near term, a c-section is generally in order. If the separation is severe, that is, if two-thirds or more of the placenta separates from the uterine wall, mom-to-be can lose up to four pints of blood—a life-threatening amount—and the situation is considered an emergency. The mother will require a rapid blood transfusion and a Cesarean will be performed immediately.

Maternal Infection with Herpes

Women who carry the herpes simplex virus (HSV)—either type 1, which causes "cold sores" on and around the face and mouth or type 2, which causes sores on and around the genitals—are at risk for passing the virus on to their newborns. Both HSV-1 and HSV-2 can be present in the birth canal, in some cases without the mother knowing it, and infection of either type is dangerous for a newborn. Babies who contract the virus at birth are at risk for brain damage or death. A 2003 study found that the longtime practice of performing a c-section on women who have active herpes dramatically reduces the odds that the newborn will become infected.

Researchers at the University of Washington compared the HSV transmission rates of 202 women who participated in the study. They found that of the women who had *active* lesions at the time of delivery, only 1 percent of the women who had Cesareans passed the virus on to their babies; 8 percent of the women who delivered vaginally gave their babies HSV.

The researchers also discovered that the women who had been infected with HSV recently (in some cases, during pregnancy) were more likely to pass on the infection, probably because their bodies had not had enough time to produce antibodies to the virus. Another finding of the study: women whose babies were monitored with scalp electrodes were more likely to transmit HSV to their babies. But Zane Brown, MD, the physician who directed the study says, "Any sort of invasive procedure used for a vaginal delivery, such as forceps or a vacuum extractor, would also increase the risk of the mother passing the virus on to her baby."

Approximately 25–33 percent of American women of reproductive age have genital herpes. Now here's the scary thing: of these, only 10 percent know that they have the infection. The other 90 percent thinks they are having recurrences of urinary tract or yeast infections, allergies to condoms or spermicides, or irritation from sex. The only way to know for certain whether or not you have HSV is to have a herpes blood test for antibodies. To be on the safe side, be sure to ask your healthcare provider to do a "*type-specific herpes antibody* test." Most labs use herpes antibody tests that are not type-specific.

Convenience for mother or physician and fears of malpractice

We know that there are plenty of pregnant women who would volunteer for scheduled Cesarean delivery—even if there were no medical reason for it. Maybe the anticipation of labor pains makes them uneasy, or perhaps they are unwilling to relinquish control of such an important event, or are worried about embarrassing themselves during labor.

In fact, elective Cesarean birth is a fast-growing trend in Mexico, Chile, and Brazil, especially among women who have private health insurance. Let us reiterate: we would never recommend this. There is a reason that women who give birth vaginally are often able to go home within twenty-four hours of giving birth, whereas women who have a Cesarean birth remain in the hospital for up to five days: it is major surgery. *Delivering a baby by Cesarean should not be taken lightly.* Still, there are physicians who will grant the mother-to-be a Cesarean if it is her wish. Of course this practice is currently frowned on by insurance companies (because of the extended hospital stay, Cesarean births are considerably more expensive than vaginal deliveries), so the physician might be forced to make up a diagnosis for Cesarean delivery.

There is evidence suggesting that physician convenience, financial incentives, and fear of malpractice contribute to the rate of Cesarean delivery in some regions. The research is contradictory, however, and, after interviewing dozens of OB/GYNs—the professionals who are responsible for the care of women at their most vulnerable and who deliver our babies—we find it hard to believe that these physicians would be cavalier about such a serious matter. When they are in the delivery room, their primary goal is to hand a healthy baby into the arms of a healthy mother.

TABLE 1: By the Numbers: Reasons Cited for Cesarean Deliveries

Repeat procedure: 87.4 percent* (the percentage of women who had a repeat Cesarean out of all the women who were eligible)

NUMBERS OF WOMEN WHO WERE DIAGNOSED WITH	PERCENTAGE OF THOSE WHO DELIVERED BY CESAREAN
Dysfunctional labor: 114,479 women**	70.7 percent
Placental abruption: 21,409	63.3 percent
Placenta previa: 13,356	81.3 percent
Cephalopelvic disproportion: 63,240	96.4 percent
Fetal distress: 140,074	61.3 percent
Genital herpes: 33,644	36.2 percent
Diabetes: 131,027	41.7 percent

* Out of 1,043,846 total Cesarean deliveries

** Out of 4,021,726 births

Martin J. A., Hamilton, B.E., Sutton, P.D., Ventura, S.I., Menacker, F., Munson, M.L., Births: Final data for 2002, National Vital Statistics Reports; Vol. 52, No. 10, Hyattsville, Maryland, National Center for Health Statistics, December 17, 2003.

Cesareans Defined

Historically, Cesareans were performed to remove a baby from a mother who had died. Today, in the majority of situations, Cesareans are performed because they are medically necessary to preserve the health of the mother, the baby, or both. A number of factors ultimately determine what kind of Cesarean a woman will have and it is helpful to understand the exact definitions. The more a woman knows about all the scenarios that might occur during pregnancy and labor, the better she will be able to make decisions that ultimately affect her own health and her baby's health.

Elective or Planned Cesarean

An elective Cesarean is one that is done for medical reasons already known to the physician during pregnancy. The surgery is scheduled before labor begins. Because the physician is already aware of the health conditions affecting the mother or fetus, the surgery can be scheduled close to the due date (unless an unforeseen scenario requires an earlier delivery date).

. . . .

Listen to your instincts

"My third pregnancy proceeded as uneventfully as my first two. Right up until thirty-five weeks. That's when we found out that Hadley was transverse. My doctor was going to wait a few days to see if she'd move into the head-down position herself before he tried to move her. But almost a week went by, Hadley hadn't budged, and one day I just didn't feel quite right. I called my doctor because I wanted him just to check and make sure everything was okay, but when I went in, we discovered that my water had broken. I had the Cesarean later that night."

—Cheryl, mother of three, one Cesarean in 2002

. . . .

Emergency or Non-elective Cesarean

When a Cesarean is performed under urgent circumstances, it is usually because something unexpected has occurred during labor or sometimes, late in pregnancy. The Cesarean is medically necessary to preserve the health—or save the lives—either of the mother, the baby, or both. Sometimes an emergency Cesarean requires a general anesthesia.

Cesarean On-Demand or Patient Choice Cesarean

In some South American countries, namely Brazil and Chile, women are increasingly requesting Cesarean deliveries even when they are not medically necessary. A surgical delivery is considered a status symbol among women in the wealthier classes, and favored by those who have private health insurance. This is a controversial issue in other countries, particularly in the United States.

In light of the rising rates of c-sections—and in response to the increasing numbers of women in the United States who are requesting elective Cesareans because they believe it will prevent future pelvic or sexual dysfunction (or because they want to avoid the pain or inconvenience of vaginal childbirth)—members of the American College of Obstetricians and Gynecologists (ACOG) Ethics Committee issued a statement about elective Cesarean in November 2003. "The evidence to support the benefit of elective Cesarean is still incomplete," reads the ACOG statement. The authors conclude that there are not enough extensive studies comparing the risk of death or illness due to Cesarean with vaginal births in healthy women. Until such studies exist, and the evidence from them suggests there is a benefit to elective Cesarean, it is unlikely that physicians in this country will routinely offer women the choice to give birth by Cesarean.

Hard Labor? It Must Be a Boy!

It's a barely kept secret among labor and delivery nurses: if there are complications during labor, odds are it's a boy. But this isn't just "an old nurses' tale" anymore; it was confirmed in a 2003 study published in the *British Medical Journal.* Researchers analyzed birth data from the National Maternity Hospital in Dublin, Ireland, looking at details from the births of 4,070 boys and 4,005 girls between 1997 and 2000. Male births were more likely to result in longer labor; with boys, mom more often required the hormone oxytocin to stimulate contractions; the boy babies required more fetal blood sampling to check on distress levels. *And boys were 30 percent more likely to be delivered via Cesarean.*

TABLE 2: A Global Perspective on Cesarean

In the United States, thanks to the quality of our health care, women are less likely to die from complications of childbirth than in most countries around the world. Maternal death remains one of the leading causes of death for women of childbearing age worldwide. But access to Cesarean deliveries is only part of the story; factors such as prenatal care also play an important role in maternal health.

According to the World Health Organization, countries in which the rate of Cesarean delivery is less than 5 percent of total birth indicate that some life-threatening complications associated with pregnancy and childbirth do not receive adequate treatment. And while the occasional network news story might lead you to believe that Cesarean rates in the United States are the highest in the world, in fact, they're not. Here's a look at Cesarean rates around the world, including maternal and neonatal mortality rates.

COUNTRY	CESAREAN RATES*	NEONATAL DEATHS PER 1000 LIVE BIRTHS 1995–2000(†)	ESTIMATED NUMBER OF MATERNAL DEATHS PER 100,000 LIVE BIRTHS 1995†
Argentina	25.4% (1996–97)	12	84
Australia	21.1% (1998)	4	6
Brazil	40% (1999)	19	262
Canada	18.7% (1997–98)	1	6
Chile	40% (1997)	38	33
China	23% (1999)	99	62
Cuba	23% (1997)	56	24
Finland	15.4% (1995)	11	6
Italy	22.4% (1995)	19	11
Japan	20% (1997)	9	12
Mexico	25% (1996)	55	67
Netherlands	9.2% (1995)	8	10
United States	26.1% (2002)	3	12

* Cesarean rates from International Cesarean Awareness Network and from a study —"Rates and Implications of Caesarean Sections in Latin America: Ecological Study"—which appeared in the *British Medical Journal*, November 27, 1999, pages 1397–1402; † Infant and maternal mortality rate statistics from Save the Children.

Where you live determines your odds of birth by Cesarean

A sampling of states with c-section rates higher than the 2002 national average of 26.1 percent*†

Alabama: 28.7 percent

Arkansas: 29.1 percent

California: 26.8 percent

Florida: 28.5 percent

Kentucky: 28 percent

Lousiana: 30.4 percent

Maryland: 27.5 percent

Massachusetts: 28 percent

Mississippi: 31.1 percent

New Jersey: 30.9 percent

New York: 27.1 percent

South Carolina: 28.6 percent

Tennessee: 27.5 percent

Texas: 27.9 percent

West Virginia: 29.3 percent

A sampling of states with c-section rates lower than 22 percent in 2002†

Alaska: 19.5 percent

Arizona: 21.3 percent

Colorado: 21.1 percent

Hawaii: 21.4 percent

Idaho: 19.7 percent

New Mexico: 19.1 percent

Utah: 19.1 percent

Vermont: 20.9 percent

Wisconsin: 20.6 percent

Wyoming: 21.1 percent

*† From National Vital Statistics Reports, Vol. 52 No. 10, December 17, 2003

A reassuring note: Dana's son, Liam, ultimately spent three weeks at the James Whitcomb Riley Hospital for Children in Indianapolis, part of the time on a respirator and heart-lung bypass machine. During labor, Liam had aspirated meconium and filled his lungs with the tarry waste that babies aren't supposed to pass until they are safely out of the womb. About 4,000 babies do the same thing each year, but most of the time physicians can suction the meconium out of the lungs before it does any damage. Thanks to his quick delivery via Cesarean, the amazing care he received as a newborn, and some wondrous technology that helped him heal, Liam is now a healthy six-year-old.

CHAPTER 2

The Surgery

There are women who give birth by Cesarean and care only to know the necessary facts, in this case, that their uterus was cut open to deliver their baby. Then there are women who, like us, become curious at some point for more details about the surgery they had days, weeks, months, or even years earlier. Or maybe you've just learned that you'll have your first c-section delivery or you're scheduling a second, third, even fourth procedure, and you have just as many questions. The following chapter takes you step-by-step through the most commonly performed surgical procedure in the United States. Having a better understanding of how the surgery is done and what your body will undergo (or underwent) will empower you as you plan for or recover from surgery.

C-Sections: The Most Frequently Performed Surgery

More than four million babies were born in the United States in 2002. And more than one million of them were delivered by c-section. While a c-section is thought of as a significant surgical procedure, most OBs consider it to be less complicated than a hysterectomy or breast augmentation. Due to the frequency with which Cesarean surgeries are performed, you can be assured that your OB's skills won't get rusty. While there are risks involved with a Cesarean, in many circumstances it is still safer for both mother and baby than forceps delivery, which used to be the only option for delivering a baby in a "dif-ficult" situation.

The Pain Patrol

It makes sense to begin with the person who will be one of the first you'll meet with as you are prepped for surgery: the anesthesiologist. This person is a medical doctor with special-ized training in anesthesiology. Her primary role is to control your pain during the procedure. Pain is managed during a c-section with one of three types of anesthesia: an epidural, a spinal block, or general anesthesia. In roughly 90 percent of c-section deliveries, an epidural and/or a spinal block is used; the remaining 8–11 percent involve general anesthesia. Epidu-rals and spinals work essentially the same way. They are both anesthetics that are injected into the fluid or tissue surrounding the spinal column to block the nerve impulses that allow you to feel from the chest down. General anesthesia is given through a combination of an IV and inhaled gases.

How Your Anesthesia Is Selected

Your anesthesiologist considers several factors before decid-ing which form of anesthesia should be administered to you:

- **The reason for the c-section.** For instance, if you are in a nonemergency situation and laboring with an epidural, the catheter is already in place in your spinal column. To prepare you for surgery, the anesthesiologist simply ups the amount of epidural to increase numbness in the lower half of your body. If you have a scheduled Cesarean delivery with no complicating factors, you're likely to get a spinal block. Spinal blocks are ideal for these situations since they provide solid pain protection for a specified amount of time. In an emergency situation there is often still time to administer a spinal or epidural. But in cases when a woman is hemorrhaging, the anesthesiologist is likely to use general anesthesia. Unlike an epidural or spinal block, a general doesn't cause a quick drop in blood pressure—something you'd want to avoid if you were hemorrhaging. Another situation that may require general anesthesia is when a baby's life is at risk and he needs to come out as quickly as possible. General anesthesia takes effect within seconds, which means that the physician can begin operating almost immediately.

- **Your current state of health.** Epidurals, for example, are preferred for women with certain types of heart problems or severe asthma. That's because an epidural numbs the body gradually, producing less of an initial shock on the system than a spinal block, which takes effect quickly and can cause a quick drop in blood pressure.

- **Your medical history.** Women who've had previous abdominal surgeries or who are obese require more time to cut through scar tissue or fatty layers. In either case, a continuous catheter-controlled epidural is a better choice than a one-shot spinal injection that could wear off in two hours.

- **Your preference as well as hers.** Barring any serious medical conditions or situations, your anesthesiologist considers your desires as well as her own preference.

The ABCs of Anesthesia

To administer a spinal block, the anesthesiologist will ask you to lie on your side or to sit up. To lessen the pain of the epidural or spinal needle, she first gives an injection of lidocaine to numb the area. (The needle containing the lidocaine is so small that it feels like a tiny pinch.)

Pros of a spinal block:
- It completely numbs from the lower chest down within about five minutes.

- Compared to an epidural, a spinal offers a better, all-over block of pain.
- It's less painful than an epidural because the needle used is smaller.
- It's easier to administer because the area on the spine is more easily located.

Cons of a spinal block:
- The effects last an average of two to four hours. For the average c-section surgery, which takes about forty-five minutes to an hour, this is more than sufficient. But if your surgery should involve complications that lengthen the procedure you won't be able to get another injection. Instead you'll be given general anesthesia to manage your pain.
- A block can cause a spinal headache. (See "The Dreaded Headache . . ." below.)
- In a small percentage of cases, the needle that administers the spinal block can cause a blood clot or an abscess, which can lead to infection. In *extremely rare* cases, temporary or permanent partial paralysis can occur due to the nerve damage.

As with the spinal, if you're getting an epidural you'll be asked to lie on your side or to sit up. A needle that holds a catheter (an elastic tube) is injected outside the dura, a tiny area outside the spinal fluid sac. Because the anesthesia isn't injected directly into the spinal fluid, it can take a little longer, about ten minutes, to achieve complete numbing of the lower body.

Pros of an epidural:
- Since the epidural anesthetic is consistently fed through a catheter that stays in place in your spine (unlike the one-time shot given for a spinal), the anesthesia lasts as long as needed for the surgery.

Cons of an epidural:

• The epidural space is a small area that sits between the bones of the back, which means it can take more than one try to accurately pinpoint the area.

• With an epidural, you're more likely to experience some sensation, like tugging or pulling, during the procedure.

• While rare, the needle that administers the epidural can cause a blood clot, or an abscess, which can lead to infection. In *extremely rare* cases, temporary or permanent partial paralysis can result due to nerve damage.

• If you do get a headache following an epidural, the pain can be quite intense.

A combination spinal-epidural, also known as a walking-epidural, can also be used for a c-section delivery. If you receive this kind of anesthesia during labor, all your doctor needs to do to prepare you for surgery is to increase the amount of epidural anesthesia being fed through the catheter.

When a patient receives general anesthesia, it's administered in two steps. First, a sedating drug is given through an IV. Then a breathing tube is inserted into your mouth and throat allowing you to inhale gases that keep you sedated. The drugs take effect within seconds and last as long as needed. The downside is that you aren't alert when your baby is born. And in rare cases serious breathing problems can occur. (See more on this, below.)

The Dreaded Headache and Other Anesthesia-Related Side Effects

A small percentage of patients who receive an epidural or spinal block will develop a nasty headache as a result, says William Camann, MD, director of obstetric anesthesia at Brigham and Women's Hospital in Boston and associate professor of anesthesia at Harvard Medical School. The reason: the tiny hole created by the needle used to administer the anesthesia in or around the spinal sac causes miniscule amounts of spinal fluid to seep out. When spinal fluid is even slightly diminished, the brain literally sags in the head. This creates pressure and pain in the head until the body has a chance to heal the hole and regenerate the fluid which takes a few days. Headaches associated with epidurals are usually more severe due to the bigger size of the catheter-needle combo required to administer them. (The larger the hole in the spinal column, the more of a chance there is for spinal fluid to leak out.)

If you experience one of these headaches, learning that the pain is due to "brain sag" can sound rather scary. But Dr. Camann explains that this is a temporary condition that rights itself even without treatment, and has no lasting effects. The real horror is the intensity of the headache and how long it can hang around: the migraine-like pain can last anywhere from two to four days. Dana was unlucky enough to suffer a postspinal anesthesia headache that lasted for three days, following the birth of her second child. "The pain was excruciating," she recalls. "It was worse than any migraine I've ever had. The throbbing literally made me stagger." She got some relief from Demerol pain medication and by lying down with her feet above the level of her head, which helped alleviate the feeling of pressure. Other treatments for a postanesthesia headache include ibuprofen or naproxen, or a blood patch that forms a clot to seal up the hole. (Even without the patch, the hole will heal itself.)

The good news is that within the last five to ten years the size of the needles used to administer spinals has gotten smaller, helping to reduce the frequency of these headaches. (Epidural needles still need to be big enough to hold a catheter.)

Other side effects from anesthesia can include blood pressure dropping too quickly, which causes the patient to faint or feel light-headed (even when lying down). The drug ephedrine is often administered intravenously to help regulate pressure.

In some cases, a patient might get an epidural or spinal block that was inadequate. When the anesthesia doesn't produce a complete block, a woman reports feeling tugging, pulling, and some pain during the procedure. For the patient with an epidural, the amount of anesthetic can be increased. The spinal is a one-shot deal, which means that the amount can't be increased. In this case, a patient feeling horrible pain would be put under with general anesthesia.

When the anesthesia's effects are too potent, you can get a claustrophobic sensation and tingling in your fingers or hands. Usually it's only the *sensation* of not being able to breathe, when in reality all of your vital signs will indicate that you are breathing just fine. If you're feeling this way, try to focus instead on nostril breathing, which can help reassure you that you are in fact getting enough air. In a small percentage of cases, the anesthesia really does go too high into the chest and interferes with breathing. If this occurs, you would be sedated and have a tube inserted down into the lungs to assist with breathing.

Breathing problems can also occur when general anesthesia is used. Though a very rare complication, a patient can cough up stomach contents that then block breathing tubes (which are routinely inserted once a patient is sedated). However, due to stricter policies on fasting before surgery, the rate of death from aspiration has declined. It's estimated that for every 10 million births, seven women die due to complications from aspiration.

The anesthesiologist may also have difficulty or be unable to insert a breathing tube for reasons such as obesity, short stature, or a blockage in the throat. But thanks to newly designed breathing tubes that are easier to insert into the airway, the number of deaths from breathing problems have been considerably reduced in the last five to ten years.

Epidural–c-section connection?

You may have heard that having an epidural during labor increases the odds of having a c-section. But the studies regarding this connection are conflicting. There does appear to be an association, but it isn't a clear case of cause and effect. A recent study, published in the July 2001 issue of *American Journal of Obstetrics and Gynecology,* found no link between epidural use and increased risk of Cesarean delivery among more than 1,000 women.

Your C-Section Team

Once it's determined which form of anesthesia you'll be getting, you are ready to head to the operating room.

If you've labored at all, you are transported on a hospital gurney. Those who've scheduled the procedure are taken by wheelchair and then asked to walk into the operating room. (Walking yourself into an operating room and then climbing up onto the table can be a very surreal experience!) Once there, a team of physicians and nurses greets you and is ready to help deliver your baby. Depending on hospital preference or policy, your c-section surgical team consists of as few as four trained staff or as many as nine. Another factor that determines how many attending surgical staff there are is the reason you're having the c-section. For example, a scheduled Cesarean with no complications won't require as many attendants as a first-time Cesarean multiple birth delivery.

Here's the rundown on the role of each primary player:

- **Primary obstetrician**—leads the surgery
- **Assisting obstetrician**—works with primary obstetrician

- **Anesthesiologist**—administers pain medication; monitors vital signs
- **Nurse or Resident anesthesiologist**—she may assist the anesthesiologist or take over once the anesthesia has taken effect
- **Scrub nurse**—hands sterile instruments to the OB
- **Circulating nurse**—handles used surgical instruments and all other activities that do not require being sterile
- **Neonatologist**—evaluates your newborn's physical condition
- **Neonatal nurse**—assists the neonatologist
- **Neonatal nurse practitioner**—assists the neonatal nurse or neonatolgist

The Nonemergency C-Section

The Preparation

- Once you are in the operating room and on the operating table, the surgical attendants begin to prep you for surgery. If an epidural isn't already in place from labor, you are asked to turn on your side to have the epidural or spinal anesthesia administered. When that's completed you are asked to lie on your back. Towels are placed under one of your hips (usually your right side) so that you aren't lying totally flat on your back. This is done to avoid compressing the vena cava vein that feeds blood and oxygen into a major heart valve and to your uterus. (It's the same reason that you're not supposed to lie flat on your back during the last trimester of pregnancy.) Some hospitals have tables that are already slightly tipped, making the towels unnecessary.
- Your partner changes into scrubs—typically a shirt and drawstring pants, a cap to cover his hair, and a sterile breathing mask.
- A nurse gives you a drink to reduce stomach acid (usually bicarbonate of citrate). This is a precautionary measure in case you ultimately need general anesthesia. In rare circum-

stances, general anesthesia causes a patient to vomit and then inhale the contents of their stomach into their lungs. The higher the acid level, the greater the risk of developing potentially fatal pneumonia or an airway blockage.

- Your pubic hair may or may not be shaved. Some hospitals have a policy to not have nurses shave expectant women's pubic hair because studies show that shaving actually increases the risk of wound infection. Shaving irritates oil glands in the skin that have infection-causing bacteria embedded in them. Some women opt to shave at home in preparation for a scheduled c-section. If you do want to shave, it's better to wait until right before the surgery since shaving pubic hair the night before allows more opportunity for bacteria to grow.

- The lower half of your belly is washed with soap to remove surface dirt and oil, and is then swabbed with antimicrobial solution, such as iodine.

- Although some hospitals will apply an antiseptic to cleanse the vaginal area before the procedure, many hospitals feel it's unnecessary and leave the area alone.

- Your nurse inserts a Foley catheter into your urinary tract to help drain urine before, during, and for about twelve to twenty-four hours following the surgery. The reason the bladder is emptied beforehand is that a full bladder is more likely to get in the way and be injured during the surgery.

- The anesthesiologist puts an intravenous line into your arm or hand so that you can receive fluids, medication, and possibly antibiotics before and throughout the procedure. Fluids are necessary because labor and/or pre-surgery dietary restrictions can dehydrate you. You also lose blood during labor and surgery. Intravenous (IV) fluids are a combination of salt water and sugar and help to expand blood volume and keep circulation going well. Your anesthesiologist also hooks you up to a monitor to measure your blood pressure, heart rate, and breathing. She'll place a tiny monitor on your index finger that checks your pulse. You are given oxygen (either through a mask or nostril tube).

- About five minutes after the anesthesia is administered, your physician checks to make sure that it's working. She might use a clamp to grab some skin to see if you feel any pinching. While it's normal to feel some sensation, experiencing pain from the pinching is an indication that the anesthesia hasn't fully taken effect or that you need more.

The Surgery

- When it's clear that the lower half of the body is numb to pain, your physician zeroes in on your lower abdomen, just above your pubic hairline. In nonemergency situations, planned or unplanned, your doctor will make a side-to-side incision in your abdomen known as the Pfannenstiel or, less formally, the bikini cut. This is a four- to six-inch lateral abdominal incision. In cases where there is a very large baby or substantial scarring from a previous Pfannenstiel incision, a cut called the Maylard may be used. This is slightly wider than the bikini cut and done an inch or so above the pubic hairline. A nonemergency c-section can also require a vertical abdominal cut. The physician may decide that a baby lying on its side is more accessible with a vertical cut, or that an obese woman may do better with a vertical because a transverse cut would be covered over by layers or fatty skin that could impede healing.

- Once the skin is cut, a tough, fibrous layer of tissue that covers the abdominal muscles is revealed. This tissue is cut laterally and then lifted off the muscle.

- It usually takes about forty-five minutes (give or take fifteen minutes) to complete a first-time Cesarean. Those who've had prior c-sections or who are obese can require more time due to extra scar tissue or fatty layers that must be cut through.

- The OB then uses her hands to separate the abdominal muscles, which run up and down.
- Underneath the abdominal muscles lies the peritoneum. The physician pokes through this layer of membrane with a scalpel, finger, or scissors to reach your uterus. To avoid damaging the bladder, which sits along the bottom of the uterus, the OB pushes it down and out of the way with her fingers or a scissors.
- At this point your physician may lay absorbent pads in the peritoneum to help soak up blood and amniotic fluid.
- Your uterus is ready to be opened. In 90 percent of all Cesarean births, a side-to-side cut called the Kerr incision is done on the lower uterus. This type of incision is preferred over a vertical because there's less bleeding and a lower risk of bladder injury or of adhesions attaching to the bowel following the surgery. The incision is made in one of two ways: your OB uses a scalpel to make a half-inch-wide cut in your lower uterus. Then, using an index finger from each hand, she stretches open the incision, making it just wide enough for the baby's head to fit through. Other physicians prefer to make an initial cut with a scalpel and then use a scissor, rather than their fingers, to further expand the incision.

  Using a scissor to widen the opening allows better control of its length, but there's the risk of more bleeding because the OB could inadvertently cut blood vessels. Meanwhile, stretching the incision manually gives less control over how far it spreads, but causes less bleeding because there's less stress put on blood vessels.

- If you are given a classic uterine incision (done in special circumstances, such as with a baby who is lying sideways or who is preterm and breech) you are cut vertically.

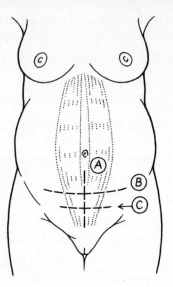

Figure 1. Three commonly used abdominal incisions: (A) Classical; (B) Maylard; (C) Pfannenstiel.

This type of uterine incision is done in just 10 percent of c-sections. It's used when quicker access and a better view of the uterus is needed. Except for a few indications, a classic incision is strongly discouraged because it causes more bleeding and puts you at higher risk of infection. In subsequent pregnancies, this type of vertical scar is also more likely to rupture than a lateral scar, putting you and your baby at risk of severe injury or death. That's why it's very important that you make sure to ask your OB which type of uterine incision you were given.

- After your uterus is cut, if your water hasn't already broken, it's ruptured with a knife, clamp, or scissor.
- Time for your baby to be born! If your baby is in the typical head-down position, your doctor slips a hand inside your uterus and cups the baby around the top of his head. In

cases of breech (feet first) or transverse lie (horizontal), the feet or tummy are grasped.

- The assisting physician then presses down on top of your uterus to help push the baby out. Once the head (or feet or buttocks) is delivered, the rest of the body follows.

- The cord is cut and clamped. Your partner may want to cut the cord at this point, but most hospitals don't allow this during a c-section because they don't want to risk contaminating a sterile area.

- After the cord is clamped, your anesthesiologist adds antibiotics to your IV to help ward off infection, oxytocin to contract your uterus and control bleeding, and, in some cases, morphine to help control pain for the next eighteen to twenty-four hours. (For more on pain relief, see Chapter Three, "Healing at the Hospital.")

- Next, the placenta is delivered and a sample of blood from the umbilical cord is taken to test for syphilis, blood sugar, and blood type. The OB then feels around inside your uterus and removes any excess membranes or placental tissue. He may use a dry cloth to wipe the inside of the uterus. Excess blood is suctioned and you are ready to be sewn up.

- Some doctors prefer to pull the uterus up and lay it outside the body so that they can see where they're stitching. (Nice visual, right?) Using something similar to a locking stitch done with knitting, your uterus is sewn from one side across with suturing thread that eventually dissolves. The same sewing procedure might be done with the skin on your stomach. The abdominal incision is covered with sterile adhesive strips and tape to help protect it while it heals over the next week or two. If your OB opts for surgical staples to close the outer layer of skin, they are removed seven to ten days following the surgery.

The unplanned vs planned

"With my first delivery I went through twenty-four hours of labor, including twelve hours of Pitocin. I was so exhausted when it finally came time for a c-section. I didn't know about the shakes from the epidural, so that freaked me out. And the incredible dryness of my mouth was awful, too. Afterward, my blood pressure shot up, so I was in recovery for a few hours, then had some other complications, which I've blessedly blocked out of my mind.

"The second time around was scheduled and a much easier experience. I was fairly rested going in, and I knew what to expect. I thought the shakes were funny this time. And the pain wasn't nearly as bad. I was up and around way before the woman in the next bed who'd delivered vaginally and had a very painful episiotomy."

—Lisa, mother of two, Cesareans in 1992 and 1996

The Emergency C-Section

In cases when a baby or mother is in danger, a vertical incision is often used on both the abdomen and uterus. This allows the OB to gain quicker and easier access to the baby. If necessary, a baby can be born in just one or two minutes once you're cut open. Since a vertical uterine incision puts you at risk for complications with future pregnancies, it's important that you know what type of incision was used with each Cesarean delivery. (For more on your incision, see Chapter Three, "Healing at the Hospital.")

The Mood in the Operating Room

Unlike the sense of urgency that prevails during an emergency c-section, the atmosphere during a nonemergency procedure can be very light, and at times even jovial. Many physicians like to play music when they operate and to chat with the patient and/or the rest of the surgical team. During one of our c-sections, the OB and attending resident went about operating while debating whether the Giants had a chance at making it to the Super Bowl. They asked if we knew the sex of the baby and whether we had settled on a name. While I (Maureen) appreciated their interest, I couldn't help but think that the lighthearted banter seemed more fitting for a cocktail party or for standing around the office water cooler! Were the doctors overlooking the serious business at hand? After talking to obstetricians who perform this surgery three or four times per week, we learned that not all surgical teams like to banter, but when they do, it's not a sign of being cavalier. In fact, one of the main reasons we're told it's done is to put the patient at ease. It's also a sign that your OB is comfortable with the task at hand and that the surgery is going well and no complications have arisen.

Despite considerable advances and improvements with Cesareans, this procedure is still considered major surgery, posing risks to both the mother and baby. One complicating factor that can be discovered during surgery is *placenta accreta*. Accreta causes certain parts of the placenta to adhere to the uterine wall, making it very difficult (or impossible) to remove the placenta. Because your obstetrician must spend additional time trying to remove the placenta, it increases the risk of blood loss and infection. If it's not possible to remove the placenta, a hysterectomy will be necessary. In other instances, women suffer injury to the bladder, kidney, uterus, or gastrointestinal tract. Often, the injury can be repaired during the procedure. However, the injury may not be apparent until after the surgery, at which point problems or infection result.

Most Cesarean-related deaths involve nonelective procedures with complications such as excessive blood loss, infection, blood clots, and problems from anesthesia. Maternal mortality associated with Cesarean delivery is estimated to be three to seven times greater than that associated with vaginal delivery. The overall mortality rate associated with Cesarean delivery is 6 per 100,000 procedures. However, when you consider only elective Cesareans involving epidural analgesia, death rates are actually lower than the mortality rates associated with all vaginal births.

For most patients, the surgery goes smoothly. And after two to three hours of monitoring in the recovery area following the operation, you're wheeled to your hospital room where you can begin your recovery.

. . . .

Relieved by her c-section

"I actually felt a sense of relief when the doctor came in and said we needed to do a c-section. I had been induced because my fluids levels around the baby were low, and I didn't get past one-and a half centimeters dilated after sixteen hours. Also, I had always been concerned about the 'engineering' aspect of vaginal delivery and was a bit scared about childbirth. I had joked that I wanted to be hit over the head with a mallet, and my section was as close as you could get."

—Christine, Cesarean in 2003

. . . .

CHAPTER 3

Healing at the Hospital

Now that you've delivered your baby, your most important task for the next few days and weeks is to give your body the rest and care it needs to heal. Thanks to the Newborns' and Mothers' Health Protection Act, a federal law enacted in January 1998, insurance companies must cover at least ninety-six hours of inpatient care following a Cesarean delivery; however most women who have an uncomplicated c-section opt to stay between forty-eight and seventy-two hours. Seeing that you've just had surgery *and* given birth, do yourself a favor and take full advantage of the time you're entitled to! Sure, after a couple of days in the hospital you'll probably be eager to get away from all the interruptions and home to your own bed. But consider that, once you're home, you likely won't have a full-time staff available to do things like change your sheets, prepare and serve you three meals a day, and bring you pain medication with a glass of water at 4:30 a.m.! While your partner, a family member, or friend will no doubt tend to your needs, they aren't going to be available twenty-four hours a day.

During your stay an obstetrician will make a daily visit to check in on you and monitor your recovery. However, a nurse trained in general obstetrics and postpartum care will oversee the bulk of your care.

Checking for Complications

For the first hour or two following your surgery you will be closely observed in a post-op recovery room. A nurse will monitor you during this period, and throughout your hospital stay, for signs of:

Uterine Infection (Postpartum Endomyometritis)

Postpartum infection is the most frequent complication with a c-section delivery. That's why some physicians prefer to give prophylactic antibiotics intravenously right before the surgery to help reduce your chances of developing a uterine infection. If you aren't given antibiotics, or the ones you were administered aren't effective at fighting off the bacteria, infection can set in within different layers of the uterus, producing symptoms about twenty-four to forty-eight hours after delivery. (However, infection can occur at any point during your recovery.) Some factors that increase your risk of developing infection include laboring prior to the surgery, having gestational diabetes, and having an emergency c-section.

Signs of infection include:
- fever
- extreme fatigue
- breathing difficulties
- abdominal pain
- uterine tenderness
- foul-smelling vaginal discharge
- chills
- change in urine volume and color

Treatment involves getting the infection under control with a stronger or a different class of antibiotics.

Excessive Blood Loss

Another complication that can develop is hemorrhaging or excessive blood loss. One doctor estimates that roughly 5–10 percent of women have excessive blood loss during or after a c-section. Even though bleeding must be under control before you leave the operating room, it can start up again at any point during recovery. The most common reason for excessive bleeding is the uterus failing to contract following the surgery. Other reasons for bleeding are cuts made on the uterus from a scalpel, a blood clot, or tiny placental parts that inadvertently weren't removed. Some conditions that increase your risk of hemorrhaging are that you had an emergency Cesarean, you labored and had surgery, you had a long Pitocin induction that was unsuccessful, or you developed a uterine infection prior to or during labor. Signs of hemorrhage include:

- a "boggy" uterus—This is a nursing term for a relaxed, enlarged uterus. Your nurse will check your uterus by placing her hands on your stomach and feeling for the fundus (the upper portion of the uterus). An enlarged fundus that is also soft instead of firm is an indication that the uterus hasn't contracted properly and is still bleeding. Uterine massage—often done every fifteen minutes for the first one to two hours, and then two to three times per day throughout your stay—can help the uterus to contract. (Even though the massage is helpful, it can be very uncomfortable because of the pressure applied near the incision.) Breastfeeding also causes uterine contractions that help the uterus get back to its original size.

- lowered blood pressure—This is often one of the first signs of excessive blood loss. When you lose large amounts of blood, you don't have the same blood volume to push against the walls of your arteries, which, in turn, causes your blood pressure to drop. As a result, you might feel light-headed, weak, and clammy.

- increased respiration and heart rate—The lack of oxygen-rich blood reaching your lungs makes breathing more difficult, which causes your heart rate and breathing to speed up.

If you show any of these signs, a doctor will be notified. In the meantime, the nurse will lower the head of your hospital bed in attempt to raise your blood pressure. You'll also be given an electrolyte solution intravenously to replace fluids and Pitocin to help contract the uterus. In extreme cases, a blood transfusion may be necessary to replenish the lost blood supply.

Wound Infection

Six to 8 percent of patients develop infection of their incision. Bacteria can invade your wound during the surgery, or be transmitted during a vaginal exam during labor or by your own hands following the surgery. Factors that increase your risk include previous incisions at the same site (which make the tissue weaker and more susceptible to infection), labor prior to the c-section, and obesity (flaps of skin cover the area, creating a moist environment for bacteria to grow). To minimize the risk of wound infections, it's common practice to give a patient intravenous antibiotics during the c-section. Traditionally, these are given right after the infant is delivered, although some doctors are now considering whether to give antibiotics prior to the initial incision to allow them more time to work. Symptoms of a wound infection aren't usually evident until three to seven days postdelivery. They include:

- redness or pain at the incision site
- fever
- bleeding or oozing from the wound

A blood culture and/or wound culture may be taken to determine the type of bacteria involved. The incision will be opened and drained and antibiotics will be given orally for several days to a week.

Blood Clots

When you're pregnant, your liver responds to the increased hormones by making more of the chemicals that cause the blood to clot. This increases your risk of blood clots, or thrombophlebitis. Having a c-section puts you at additional risk because lying in bed for extended periods can cause blood to pool and form clots.

A clot can develop at any time following the surgery and for up to approximately six months afterward. Compared to those who deliver vaginally, c-section patients are three to five times more likely to develop clots. Patients at highest risk include those who are very obese, patients who had a difficult surgery with excessive bleeding, women with a uterine infection prior to their c-section, and those with a history of blood clots. A clot typically starts in the deep veins of the legs. If one travels to the lungs, it can block the pulmonary artery (the vein that pumps blood to your lungs), causing death.

Symptoms of a blood clot include:
- isolated pain in the lower legs
- swelling and redness in the affected area

To prevent clots you are urged to get up and start moving within twelve to twenty-four hours following the surgery (or sooner, if you are up to it), and to take short walks a few times each day while in the hospital. While in bed, make a point every hour to bend your knees, flex your legs, and rotate your ankles. Some hospitals have high-risk patients wear elasticized stockings because the squeezing pressure on the legs increases circulation. Treatment for a blood clot includes an intravenous blood thinner such as Heparin, to help break up the clot. Once you leave the hospital you'll be given a blood thinner medication, such as Coumadin, to take orally for several weeks.

Reaction to Anesthesia

If you've had general anesthesia you can feel nauseous or may vomit as the medication wears off. Very often, women who receive an epidural or spinal will experience uncontrollable shivering known as "the shakes." These are completely harmless, and though they can start in the operating room, you're more likely to develop them in the recovery room as the anesthesia wears off. Your nurse may cover you in warm blankets and administer warm IV fluids to try to minimize them. If the shaking is extreme, some physicians will give a narcotic such as Demerol to control the shaking.

Although it's not standard practice yet, some hospitals have begun giving patients a dose of morphine through the epidural or spinal toward the end of the surgery to help control postsurgery pain. The effect lasts for eighteen to twenty-four hours and does an amazing job at keeping patients comfortable following abdominal surgery. One downside is that morphine can cause minor to intense, all-over itching. This is not an allergic reaction to the drug but an unfortunate side effect. If it becomes intolerable, a narcotic such as Nubain can be given to help control the itching. An antihistamine such as Benadryl can also be used.

To make sure that you're regaining sensory awareness, the nurse will ask you to wiggle your toes and if you can feel your legs. (It's a very odd sensation when you reach down and feel partially numb legs!) Your nurse is making sure that you're getting feeling back on both sides of the body. Full feeling returns on average in about four hours following the surgery.

In *extremely rare* cases, a spinal or epidural anesthesia can damage a nerve in the spinal column, causing partial paralysis. The paralysis is usually due to nerve damage that results from a blood clot or infection at the site of the injection. To give you some idea of how infrequently this occurs, an anesthesiologist from Brigham and Women's Hospital in Boston—where 10,000 babies are delivered each year—said that in his twenty year career he's never once seen a case of permanent paralysis from regional anesthesia used for a delivery.

Injury or Infection of Bladder or Urinary Tract

Since the bladder lies over the lower portion of the uterus, it must be pushed aside to deliver baby via c-section. This can result in a nick in the bladder which can allow bacteria to invade. The Foley catheter is another transmitter for bacteria. Your nurse will monitor you for signs of infection or injury that include:
- a drop in urine output
- blood-tinged urine
- pain or pressure when you urinate

You'll be treated with antibiotics.

Side Effects from Labor and Pushing

If you've labored for any length of time *and* had a c-section, having to deal with additional side effects like vaginal swelling, tearing, and hemorrhoids is no picnic. Your nurse will assess your injuries and apply an ice pack to treat swelling and tears. You'll also be given Proctocream (25 percent hydrocortisone) and pads coated with witch hazel to help reduce hemorrhoidal swelling.

Vaginal Bleeding

Whether you've labored or not before your c-section, you will still experience a menstrual-like blood flow from your vagina for about a month or so afterward. While the flow is generally lighter than that of those who've delivered vaginally (a uterus that doesn't have an incision contracts better, thereby causing more blood to be expelled), expect some days to be heavier than others. The color will also change, usually from brownish-red to reddish to pink. Extremely heavy bleeding (bleeding that requires changing your pad every hour) is not normal and should be checked by your obstetrician.

One of the pluses to delivering by c-section is that there is less strain put on the vagina, as well as the urinary tract, bowels, and perineum (the area between the vagina and rectum). Some studies indicate that those who deliver by c-section may have fewer incidences of painful sex, urinary and fecal incontinence, or a pelvic-organ prolapse (a condition that requires surgery to repair). Other studies show that the damage to these areas may occur during pregnancy, which means that how you deliver may not be a factor.

Post-Op Recovery: Don't Go It Alone

Even if you're alert following the surgery, not all hospitals allow a newborn to accompany his mother to the recovery room. Instead, hospital procedure may require that the baby head straight to the nursery, where he can be warmed or given his first bath. Not wanting your partner to miss out on all the firsts, you might insist that he go with the baby. But then you're left in the recovery room all by your lonesome. If you're scheduled for the surgery, find out about the hospital's policy in advance. If they don't routinely allow newborns to accompany mom into the recovery room, ask if they make exceptions. If the answer is still no, arrange to have another family member or close friend sit with you so you don't feel so alone.

Room Check-In

Once you're given the green light to leave the recovery area, you'll be wheeled to your room. Because you may still be feeling groggy and tired from the stress of the surgery, blood loss, and anesthesia, the nurses will help move you to your bed.

Many hospital maternity wards now offer private rooms in addition to their double rooms. These single rooms are usually assigned on a first-come, first-served basis.

If you must share a room, there are pluses and minuses to being paired up with a fellow c-sectioner or a vaginal birther. If you're put in a room with a woman who had c-section delivery, what better person to offer you moral support than someone who's been through the same experience as you have? I [Maureen] recalled trying in vain *and pain* late one night to move from my back to my side in the hope of finding a more comfortable position. Through the curtain that separates roommates came a concerned voice asking, "You okay? I know, the pain can be pretty awful at first." Then, when my roommate was having trouble nursing the next morning because she couldn't find a comfortable position, I was happy to be able to share a few tips I'd learned from breast-feeding my first son after surgery. The downside to this arrangement is that you'll both have constant interruptions (blood-pressure readings, temperature and incision checks, pain medication drop-offs) required for c-section patients. This can mean that neither of you gets much sleep. Meanwhile, if your roommate delivered vaginally, it can be kind of hard to watch how easy it is for her to get around mere hours after the birth (though we know very well that not all vaginal birthers are popping out of bed soon after and many are in quite a bit of pain postpartum).

No matter what your room situation your first priority should be to get the rest and care you need for recovery. Since part of your care involves very close monitoring of your overall health, expect regular visits throughout the day and night.

With each visit your nurse will do a head-to-toe assessment to check:

- **your general state**—She'll note things like whether you're awake and oriented or sleepy.
- **breathing and respiration**—She'll use a stethoscope to listen to heart and lung sounds; she'll take your blood pressure.
- **bowel sounds**—The stress of the surgery and general anesthesia slow up your bowels. Your nurse will use a stethoscope to listen for movement of the bowels (a sign that your intestines are beginning to work efficiently again); she'll ask if you're passing gas or if you've moved your bowels.
- **how much you're urinating**—Too little urine could signal dehydration or infection.
- **for blood clots**—She'll ask if you have any pain in your legs and she'll observe your legs for redness.
- **for side effects from laboring**—If you've labored, the nurse will ask you to roll on to your side so she can examine your rectum for hemorrhoids and your perineum for any bleeding or tearing.
- **your sanitary pad**—She'll make sure your vaginal bleeding isn't extremely heavy.
- **the incision**—She'll make sure there are no tears or signs of infection.

Take a Deep Breath

Starting from day one, you should try to do some deep breathing exercises as you rest in your bed. Breathing deeply will help cleanse your lungs of residual anesthesia and reduce risk for postoperative respiratory difficulties. Aim for doing these simple exercises several times a day:

- **diaphragmatic breathing**—While lying flat on your back, place your hands or a pillow over your incision. Take a series of deep breaths so that your entire abdomen—not just your lungs—expands. Repeat six to eight times.

- **lower chest expansion**—Rest your hands on the lower part of your rib cage. Take a deep breath, and focus on trying to expand your lungs under your hands. Repeat six to eight times.
- **upper chest expansion**—Rest your hands on the upper part of your rib cage. Take a deep breath, and focus on trying to expand your lungs under your hands. Repeat six to eight times.

Staying Clean

A nursing assistant will give you a sponge bath and change your sanitary pads until you are able to use the bathroom and shower unassisted. You'll also be provided with a basin so you can brush your teeth and wash your face and hands in bed.

By day two or three you'll probably feel up to showering. Since you'll be standing and moving more than usual, make sure your pain medication is working and that you don't feel weak or lightheaded before getting in the shower. (It might help to eat a small snack or meal about half an hour before doing this type of physical exertion. Fluids are also very important for energy.) Take it slow in the shower. Use the small stool they provide or the bars on the walls to maintain your balance. It's fine to get the incision area wet and soapy. Just be sure to rinse it well and then pat the area dry (moist areas can harbor bacteria). Do not apply powder or cream to the incision area. *(See below for more tips on incision care.)*

Pass the Pain Meds, Pleeeze

Your abdomen and uterus have just been cut open—even with medication to manage your pain you can definitely count on being uncomfortable for a while. Controlling pain should be your first order of business. By this we mean making sure you don't get to the point where you're yelling out in the middle of the night for your pain meds. If you got a dose of morphine with your epidural or spinal, or an injection, this will do an amazing job of controlling pain for eighteen to twenty-four hours following your surgery. (Unfortunately, in addition to itching, another possible side effect of morphine is nausea and vomiting.)

If you didn't get morphine, you'll get the next best thing: a patient-controlled anesthesia (PCA) pump. The intravenous pump contains a narcotic such as Demerol or morphine. The pump allows you to administer pain medication as you need it, giving you more control over your pain. If you had general anesthesia, the PCA pump is ideal because you are unable to take anything by mouth—even a pain pill—for a specified period of time. In hospitals that don't offer the pump, patients who've had general anesthesia will need to get multiple injections to control pain for the first twenty-four hours, sometimes followed by pain medication in pill form. Those who've had an epidural or spinal will also take oral pain medication following their surgery if the pump is not available.

Very little of these drugs passes through breast milk, so they are considered safe for your baby. (One side effect is that the baby may be more sleepy as a result.) The physical stress of a c-section surgery can reduce the production of the hormones oxytocin and prolactin, which are needed to produce breast milk. "Staying ahead of your pain," as the nurses like to say, can help reduce these effects.

Controlling pain is key to your overall recovery as well: when you feel pain you don't sleep well, you don't feel like moving, or breast-feeding. That's why it's important to take your next dose of pain medication before the previous dose has had a chance to fully wear off. When the pain medication is working the way it should, it's very easy to be fooled into thinking you don't need that next dose. Then, BAM, the pain hits you like a ton of bricks and you're running (or rather walking very slowly) for your bed. But this isn't the time to tough it out. If you know you get your medication every three hours, and you haven't seen the nurse, don't hesitate to ring for her.

Percocet is the narcotic many hospitals give to Cesarean section patients. Percocet is a combination of the narcotic oxycodone and the analgesic acetaminophen. The drug slows the central nervous system which helps block the sensation of pain. Very little of it gets into breast milk and what does will not harm your baby. When taken in large doses or for long periods of time, Percocet can be addictive. So follow your doctor's instructions on how much and for how long you should take the drug. While Percocet offers great pain protection, this medication does have side effects, though they are usually mild. The drug can make your head feel cloudy or cause dizziness, as well as cause dry mouth, itching, nausea, weakness, and constipation. (Of all of these possible side effects, constipation is probably the last thing you need when your bowels are already struggling to work! A stool softener, such as Colace, which hospitals routinely give following a c-section, can help lessen this effect from the medication.)

By day two or three you should be ready to take a less potent painkiller like ibuprofen. This provides good pain control and avoids many of the narcotic side effects such as constipation. But since ibuprofen can be tough on your stomach, it's wise to take it with a light snack or a small meal. Some hospitals are allowing c-section patients to administer their own over-the-counter medications. Called Bedside SAM (Self-Administered Medications), it provides each patient with little bottles that sit at their bedside, giving them more control in managing their pain and recovery. SAM includes a stool softener (Colace), ibuprofen (Motrin), and acetaminophen (Tylenol) to take as needed.

Despite the pain medication, movement of any kind (from coughing, laughing, sneezing, nursing, or changing positions in bed) is likely to be very uncomfortable. It can help to hold a small pillow gently over the incision site to stabilize it.

Getting Out of Bed for the First Time

Even with assistance and painkillers, getting out of bed the first few times after a c-section surgery can be very difficult. Most nurses encourage you to try to get out of bed within twelve to twenty-four hours following the surgery, if not sooner. In addition to pain, many women report feeling the sensation that their insides are falling out. Rest assured, they are not—you've been stitched back together! The sensation is due to the fact that a surgeon has cut or separated every lining in your abdomen to get to your baby. You feel the weight of the separation. These weakened areas need time to heal.

Just remind yourself that there's a good reason to be motivated to move: it helps prevent or reduce the buildup of painful gas, and lessens your risk for blood clots and pneumonia. Have your partner or a nurse assist you as you try to move about. At first, your only goal should be going from your bed to a chair. You can work up to moving about the room, and eventually you'll be ready for short walks up and down the hallway of the maternity wing.

Because you'll be weak from the surgery and still on judgment-impairing medication, someone should help you the first few times you pick up your newborn. Then, depending on how you feel and how much medication you're on, you may want to ask for help and have the nurse or your partner bring your baby to you as you sit in a chair or on your bed to nurse or bottle-feed him.

What You Must Know About Your Incision

When you undergo a c-section, your OB makes two incisions: one in your abdomen and the other in your uterus. They are not always the same kind of cut. Since the type of incision made on your *uterus* will affect future pregnancies, it's important that you know whether it was a *vertical* or *transverse* cut. Reasons a vertical uterine cut may be necessary include delivering a baby who is extremely large or lying sideways (transverse). Because a vertical incision is larger, it takes longer to heal. Even when it does heal, there is scar tissue that is never as strong as the muscles of the uterus. A vertical cut also affects the upper part of the uterus and causes weakening of a muscular area that helps to expel a fetus during a vaginal delivery. For both these reasons, a vertical uterine incision is more likely to rupture in future pregnancies and deliveries. That's why it's critical that you know what kind of incision you have and that your doctor note it in your medical records. You'll also be monitored more closely throughout future pregnancies. Women who are at a higher risk for uterine rupture may have the surgery scheduled earlier than usual, at around thirty-seven or thirty-eight weeks.

Due to the risk of uterine rupture associated with previous vertical uterine incision, ACOG recommends that all subsequent pregnancies be delivered by c-section.

Incision Care

Beyond washing and drying the incision area just as you would any other area of your body, there's no extra care that needs to be taken. If you have had a transverse incision and been closed with staples they'll be removed within three to four days. If you have had a vertical incision and staples they can come out in seven to ten days. If you were stitched up, the stitches dissolve and are absorbed internally and the bandage will come off on its own.

As with any skin wound, be sure to wash your hands thoroughly before touching the incision area so that you don't transmit germs that can lead to infection.

You can expect the incision area to be quite sore and painful for at least a week or so. Gradually, it'll taper off to a tenderness, and eventually, when you're well on you're way to being healed, the area will feel itchy on and off for a period. Occasionally some women also feel numbness or at times a tugging sensation.

Signs of infection include: warmness around the area, red streaks, bleeding, or oozing from the incision. Call your doctor right away if you notice any of these symptoms.

Those Oh-So-Horrendous Gas Pains

For some women, the pain from a uterine contraction or an abdominal incision doesn't come close to the gut-wrenching spasms that result when large amounts of air get trapped in your intestines following a c-section. One of us had such bad gas pains that she was forced to get up within only a few hours of the surgery to walk the hospital hallways for long stretches of time in hope of getting some relief. Movement is the number-one remedy for getting the gas to work its way out of your system. Your nurse will use a stethoscope to listen to bowel sounds. You'll also be given regular doses of simethicone, an anti-gas medication, and Colace, a stool softener. If the gas gets really backed up, you can request a rectal suppository for relief.

If you're scheduled for the surgery, you can try to minimize the gas pains with a presurgery diet. Forty-eight hours before the surgery, start a semiliquid diet. A yogurt or pasta soup is much easier for the intestines to digest than a cheeseburger and French fries. Some other good choices include Jell-O, eggs, and pudding.

Instead of lying flat on your back in bed for long periods (which traps gas), do yourself a favor and try to change positions at least every hour (even if it's as subtle as bending your knee, leaning to one side, or placing a pillow under one buttock).

Passing gas for the first time following a c-section is a definite cause for celebration. First, it helps relieve that horrible pressure in your stomach and, second, it's a sign that your bowels are finally moving things along. Your first bowel movement can offer the same kind of relief. But be warned that while the actual passing of stool shouldn't be painful, it can be very uncomfortable to sit on the toilet and use your stomach muscles to push.

Comforts from Home

Having a few personal items with you during your hospital stay can give your spirits a lift and make your stay more tolerable. If you're scheduled for the surgery, you can pack these items ahead of time; otherwise, have your partner bring them to you during one of his visits.

- **Personal pillow(s).** There's nothing more comforting while you're in the hospital than having a pillow from home covered in a super-soft pillowcase.
- **Comfortable clothing.** After the first day, you can ditch your hospital gown for a cotton nightgown or a pair of loose-fitting lightweight cotton pajamas or T-shirt and boxer shorts. Avoid elastic waist bottoms (a drawstring waist is perfect) because you don't want any added pressure on your stomach area. A button-down top is more convenient if you still have an IV or are nursing. Avoid long nightgowns. One that hits your knees can get twisted in bed, making it difficult to move around—the last thing you need to deal with. And, of course, don't forget a robe and a pair of slippers to put on once you're ready to get up and moving.
- **Hair accessories.** Since you won't be washing your hair for a day or more, a hair clip, tie, or band will come in handy.
- **Prescription glasses.** Having to put in contacts can be a bother when you're in the hospital. And hospital air tends to be dry, which can irritate eyes wearing contacts.
- **Makeup and earrings.** You can't underestimate the feel-

good effect you get from applying a bit of lipstick and eye makeup or from wearing earrings while you're laid up.

- **Toiletries.** Cost-cutting requirements have forced many hospitals to do away with such amenities as toothbrushes, toothpaste, and shampoo in the maternity ward. Also pack some hand sanitizer and moisturizing lotion since you'll want to clean your hands frequently.

- **A CD or cassette headset.** The maternity ward can be a noisy place. Listening to some relaxing music on a headset is a great way to tune out your roommate, her visitors, or a baby crying down the hall.

"The most unpleasant part of my hospital stay was not really getting any rest for five days because of all the noise and sleep interruptions."
—Judy, mother of two boys, both born by c-section, in 1998 and 2000

- **A framed family photo.** When you're not feeling so hot, it's nice to be able to glance over at a photo of you with your husband and any older children. If an older child has sent you a homemade card or picture, hang it on the wall (along with any other congratulatory cards you may have received). Many hospitals have small bulletin boards near the patient's bedside for this very purpose.

- **Aromatherapy oils.** Soothe yourself by dabbing on some stress-reducing lavender oil or spritzing your pillow with the sweet scent of orange or vanilla.

Top Patient Mistakes

We spoke to a registered nurse who is head of obstetrics at St. Barnabas Hospital in Livingston, New Jersey, which has one of the busiest labor and delivery units in the country. Her hospital averages 8,000 newborn deliveries a year. We asked her for advice on how c-section patients could make the most of their hospital stay. She said that without realizing it, too often women do little things that wind up having a negative impact on their recovery.

She polled the nurses on her staff and they came up with the six most common "mistakes" recovering c-section patients make during their hospital stay:

Too Many Visitors and Phone Calls

The birth of a baby is no doubt one of the highpoints in a woman's life. Understandably, you can't wait to share the good news with family and friends. But it's important to remember that along with birthing a baby, you've also just undergone surgery. Your body is tired and needs to rest. And whether you realize it or not, a steady flow of well-meaning visitors can be a drain on you. If you feel overwhelmed by the number of visitors, don't hesitate to politely ask if your neighbor or co-worker wouldn't mind putting off her visit until you are home. If you're feeling tired, let your visitors know that you'd like to take a short nap. They can use the time to visit the baby at the nursery or grab a cup of coffee with your partner. Phone calls can also be an intrusion after a while. If you're getting worn down from all the well-wishers, have your husband answer the phone, or better yet, turn it off when you know you'll be sleeping.

Touching Your Incision Without First Cleaning Your Hands

Initially, your incision is going to be sore and painful while it heals. And while your nurse will encourage you to do daily checks—for bleeding, oozing, infection—it's essential that your hands be clean before touching the area. Otherwise, you risk transmitting bacteria that can lead to infection. If you're not up to a trip to the bathroom to wash your hands, a hand sanitizing lotion or wipe will suffice.

Not Getting Up Soon Enough or Often Enough

Sometimes patients resist getting out of bed for fear of the pain. But getting your body up and moving is important for several reasons. For one, ACOG says that walking is the best way to reduce your chances of developing a life-threatening blood clot. Moving around will also prevent or reduce the build-up of painful abdominal gas, and it lowers your chance of developing pneumonia (a risk due to the anesthesia that is still in your lungs).

Before attempting to get out of bed, make sure you have a nurse to assist you in case you feel weak or lightheaded. During the first twenty-four hours following the surgery you should attempt to get up at least twice for a ten to twenty minute period. Try for three to four times on the following day. What you do while you're resting is just as important: when in bed, flex your feet, bend your knees, lift your legs, move from side to side, and take nice deep breaths.

Failing to Ask for Help with Breast-feeding

Breast-feeding is a learned skill. Nursing following a c-section can be a challenge. At most large hospitals, there are nurses available around the clock who are specially trained to assist new mothers with nursing. Take advantage of their knowledge. Even if it's 2:15 a.m., there's no reason why you should feel uneasy about buzzing for help. Starting out right and feeling confident about what you're doing are both key to successful breast-feeding.

Allowing Your Pain Medication to Wear Off

When you're feeling good thanks to pain medication, it's easy to think you can do without it. But when you don't take pain medication, you can pretty much count on feeling lousy. And when you feel lousy, you slow up your recovery because you can't sleep, and you don't want to eat or walk around. It'll also be uncomfortable to hold your newborn. (Not to mention that not sleeping or eating can affect your milk supply.) Taking your pain medication at regular intervals, before the previous dose has a chance to wear off, will allow you to stay ahead of the pain.

Eating Solid Foods Too Soon

Your bowels need time to recover from the stress of the surgery. It could be a few days before things are moving along in your intestines at a normal speed. But just because you've passed gas or had your first bowel movement doesn't mean it's time for McDonald's. Do your intestines a favor, and take it *slow*. Your nurse will guide you on what to eat when. Many hospitals now allow a full diet within hours of the surgery. But be careful when selecting your solids: foods too high in fiber, such as a bran muffin or salad, can create gas, as can carbonated beverages and chocolate. Other hospitals go by the rule that you should have nothing by mouth for the first twelve to twenty-four hours, followed by a diet with clear liquids like Jell-O, broth, or apple juice. If you tolerate those well, you can start with semisolids such as pudding, yogurt, or soup with pasta before attempting solids like a muffin or bagel.

CHAPTER 4

Your C-Section Baby

When pregnancy reaches its natural conclusion, a series of steps take place that trigger labor. The onset of labor is a delicate dance and the most important step is initiated by the baby. When a fetus has neared the end of its development, it sends a signal to the placenta—in the form of chemicals called catecholamines, also known as "stress" or "fight or flight" hormones—that it is ready for "birth day." Even though catecholamines are generally referred to as stress hormones, in birthing it might be better to consider them "excitement" hormones. Essentially, the fetus is excited because he's ready to be born and the presence of these hormones helps him adapt to life outside the womb.

Catecholamines perform other functions as well. At the onset of labor, the hormones send blood away from "nonessential" organs, such as the skin, in order to keep the essential ones, e.g., the brain and heart, well supplied with blood and oxygen.

Babies who are delivered vaginally experience another surge in catecholamines that, among other things, helps them deal with potential oxygen deprivation during birth. Babies who are delivered via Cesarean, without experiencing any labor, have much lower levels of these hormones present at birth. The presence of catecholamines before and during labor leads some health-care providers to believe that Cesareans shouldn't be scheduled prior to the natural onset of labor.

Catecholamines also help absorb amniotic fluid from the lungs, and they stimulate the production of surfactant in the lungs. Surfactant is a slippery substance that keeps the lungs surfaces from sticking together and prevents them from collapsing once the baby is outside the womb and breathing air. Some physicians speculate that because this cascade of events doesn't take place in Cesarean-born babies, it is one reason that some have difficulty breathing at first. Plus, even with all the technology we have—from sonograms that measure the baby's size to amniocentesis that can be used to check lung development—babies occasionally get delivered by Cesarean too soon. When that happens, the baby can face a host of problems associated with incomplete lung development and prematurity.

If you know in advance that you are going to deliver by Cesarean—and neither you nor your baby is experiencing any difficulties—you may want to discuss with your physician the pros and cons of waiting for labor to begin naturally rather than scheduling the surgery on an arbitrary day.

Why bother, you ask? After all, isn't one of the benefits of a scheduled Cesarean delivery skipping the labor pains? Well, a number of studies suggest that if the baby initiates labor and then experiences some pre-Cesarean contractions, he may benefit from the natural hormones discussed above. One study in particular found that full-term babies who experienced labor before a Cesarean delivery were 20 percent less likely to experience respiratory difficulties than the babies who'd been delivered via elective Cesarean prior to the onset of labor. It should be noted that waiting for labor to begin does put a woman at higher risk of infection following a c-section. Also, if you have a full stomach, and then require general anesthesia, you risk serious breathing problems associated with aspirating stomach contents. For this reason your obstetrician may be reluctant to honor your request. Another option is to request that your Cesarean not be done until the thirty-ninth week. A British study that examined nine years of birth records—some 33,000 babies—compared the rates of respiratory illness among babies who were delivered by elective Cesarean during Week 37 and those who delivered during Week 39. The babies born during Week 39 were less likely to experience respiratory problems.

The First Minutes Following Delivery

You've waited patiently for months to meet this little person and now suddenly here he is. Even if his birth didn't unfold quite the way you'd expected, meeting your newborn for the first time is likely to be one of the most memorable moments of your life. Assuming that the only real complication associated with your baby's birth is his mode of delivery, you can expect what happens next to be virtually the same as if he'd been born vaginally.

Immediately after he is born, the birth attendants will observe your baby to see how he is coping with life outside the womb. While you're being stitched up, nurses and possibly a pediatrician or neonatologist (a physician who specializes in caring for newborns) are assessing your baby's breathing, skin tone, heart rate, and other functions that indicate how he's doing (see "A Newborn's First Important Test," page 70). Before you leave the operating room, a nurse will also measure the diameter of your baby's head and his height from head to toe. She'll run a finger inside his mouth to check for a cleft palate and she'll probably jiggle his hips to make sure they're not dislocated. Your newborn will also be weighed and all his statistics recorded for his birth record.

What A Newborn Looks Like

When you gaze at your newborn, you'll notice the color of his hair and eyes, the shape of his nose, and the curve of his mouth. Since his head wasn't pressed and squeezed to fit through the birth canal, it will likely be a lovely round shape. If you did labor and push, you may notice some lumps and bumps that you didn't expect. But of course your baby will still be the most beautiful creature you've ever seen. Among the things that you perhaps didn't expect to observe, but that are entirely normal:

- **A creamlike coating covering baby's skin.** Known as *vernix,* this sometimes thick substance forms a protective coating on baby's skin. It will be absorbed into the skin so it's not necessary to wipe off except in the folds of the arms and legs, the groin and neck, and from the hair.

- **Dark hair covering large parts of baby's body.** *Lanugo* is hair that sometimes covers parts of a newborn's face and body. If the baby is premature, he may be nearly covered in it. Lanugo generally falls off within a few weeks of birth.

- **A blisterlike bump on baby's head.** If you experienced some labor before your Cesarean, your baby may have been born with an obvious bump on his head. This bump, called a *caput succedaneum,* formed when his head was pushing down on your cervix before the second stage of labor. The caput does not affect the baby's brain and will disappear within a few days.

- **Blue patches on baby's tummy or back.** These spots—known as *Mongolian spots*—alarmingly resemble bruises, and are relatively common in babies born to parents of African, Asian, Indian, or Mediterranean descent. They occasionally appear in babies who are light-skinned. These patches generally disappear by baby's first birthday.

- **Very obvious sexual characteristics.** It's typical for premature babies to have startlingly enlarged genitals. There may also be milk in the breasts of both girls and boys, and sometimes baby girls bleed vaginally. None of this is anything to worry about; it's the result of the drop in estrogen that the baby received during pregnancy, and things will look closer to scale within a few weeks.

A Word About Bonding

A frequent frustration that women who deliver via Cesarean experience is the inability to be left alone with their partner to hold and snuggle their newborns within minutes of delivery. During pregnancy and in childbirth education classes, we hear so much about the importance of establishing an immediate bond with our newborn. If the circumstances of your Cesarean mean you're unable to hold your baby as soon as he's born, you may feel like you have somehow failed in this all-important endeavor.

If your baby has some difficulties, such as needing extra oxygen, or requires observation by a nurse or neonatologist, you may in fact have to wait a little while until you can see him (though in most cases your partner will be able to accompany the baby to the special care nursery). If the Cesarean was done under emergency circumstances, and you required general anesthesia, it could be several hours before you and your baby can meet for the first time. If the baby is born with problems that require medical intervention, it will likely be much longer than that. One of us didn't get to hold her baby for the first time until he was a week-and-a-half old. Does that mean our attachment is somehow less strong than that of the baby who was in his mother's arms a few seconds after birth? Absolutely not!

Bonding is a process that takes weeks and months and years. It is most certainly not a now-or-never situation. To us, bonding means getting to know and love your baby—and it's what you'll do naturally. If for any reason you can't hold or be with your baby right after your Cesarean, you must not blame yourself, or feel like you are shortchanging your baby. Some situations are beyond your control. And keep in mind, many women who have vaginal births may also need to be separated from their babies.

If, however, you do have the opportunity to snuggle with your baby immediately—while your incision is being stitched up—we highly recommend it. You've waited months for this meeting. Because your arms will likely be restrained, and you'll have the IV in for about twenty-four hours following surgery, you will need assistance from your partner and/or a nurse. Don't be shy about asking for help. If you plan to breast-feed, this is a time that you can put your baby to breast, but don't worry if he doesn't actually latch on (again, you will need help with this and shouldn't be reluctant to request it). Just let him look at you and learn your scent and voice.

This is also an ideal time for your partner to do what you can't. He should take the opportunity to cuddle and talk softly to the baby, and if the baby needs to go to the nursery for any follow-up care, your partner should certainly go along (though you may prefer that he stay by your side). Unless it is medically necessary for your baby to be away from you, you may request that once you are out of recovery, he be brought to your room for the duration of your stay if the hospital allows room-sharing. Spending lots of time with your newborn, even during these early days when you're likely to be uncomfortable, will give you time to concentrate on those loving, mothering, feelings that may have been absent on the heels of your delivery. (However, you should not feel guilty about choosing to have your baby sleep in the nursery for certain periods. These little breaks will allow you to catch up on rest so that you regain the strength you'll need for when you go home.)

A Newborn's First Important Test

One minute after delivery, your baby will be assessed and given a score based on how he is responding to life in his new world. Then the test will be repeated after five minutes. Usually a baby who has a low score the first time will get a "better" score the second time around. Physicians use the APGAR scale to gauge a baby's initial health, based on factors such as his skin tone and his facial expressions. A "perfect" APGAR score is a ten, but a baby who scores a seven is considered healthy. A baby whose score is zero to three needs resuscitation and babies with scores in the middle, four to six, may require various interventions, including extra oxygen.

POINTS GIVEN:		0 POINTS	1 POINT	2 POINTS
A	Activity and muscle tone	Limp	Some motion of extremities	Active motion
P	Pulse rate	Absent	Below 100 beats per minute	Above 100 beats per minute
G	Grimace (response to catheter inserted in nostril)	No response	Grimace	Cough or sneeze
A	Appearance; skin color	Blue or pale	Extremities blue and body pink	Pink all over
R	Respiration	Absent	Slow, irregular	Regular, crying

Some Possible Risks for Babies Born via Cesarean

A word of warning: the information that follows pertains only to babies who must spend time in the Neonatal Intensive Care Unit (NICU) or Intensive Care Nursery (ICN) and includes information that you may find disturbing. *The majority of babies who are born via Cesarean do not need special care*, so we would suggest that you skip this section unless you need it.

As we discussed earlier, babies who are delivered by Cesarean are more likely to experience breathing difficulties than babies who are born vaginally. In fact, a recent study found that babies born by elective Cesarean are five times more likely to experience respiratory diseases than babies born vaginally. One condition that can affect either full term or premature infants is called "transient tachypnea of the newborn" and it simply means that the baby's lungs were not able to absorb all of the fluid that was present in his lungs while he was in utero. One explanation for this is the absence of the catecholamine surge. (See the beginning of this chapter for a detailed explanation.) Babies who have transient tachypnea often show signs of breathing difficulty, including grunting with each breath, and they may also appear slightly blue from lack of oxygen. In this case they may require oxygen, but the condition usually clears up within about three days of delivery.

One of the more extreme breathing difficulties that babies born via Cesarean face is called respiratory distress syndrome (RDS), or hyaline membrane disease, and it can be life-threatening. (Besides being more common in Cesarean-born babies than in babies born vaginally, RDS also affects babies born prematurely, babies born to mothers who have diabetes, and multiples.) Respiratory distress syndrome occurs when a baby's lungs are not able to function well enough to sustain the baby after his birth. Babies with RDS are kept in the NICU where, among other treatments, they are kept warm, which minimizes their need to use oxygen to maintain their body temperature. Babies with RDS usually need supplemental oxygen and sometimes must be put on a ventilator. The babies are also given surfactant, which helps their lungs function properly.

Special Situations: Babies Who Need Extra Care

If your baby is born prematurely, or has other medical problems at birth, he will probably be transferred to the hospital's NICU. This is a hospital unit where the staff is trained to meet the unique needs of newborns who are ill. If your hospital doesn't have a NICU, and your baby requires certain kinds of medical attention, he may be transferred to another hospital that has the equipment and the special staff that he needs.

The unique challenges your baby faces will determine the scope of his care. At the very least you can expect to meet a neonatologist who will head up the team who will care for your baby. The team may also include a neurologist, a cardiologist, a respiratory therapist (a specialist who administers treatments that help with breathing), a pharmacist, a nutritionist, and perhaps a pediatric surgeon. We know from firsthand experience that people who choose to attend to ailing newborns are among the kindest and most devoted people you will ever meet. And they want be as helpful as they can in what is always a very difficult situation. They will patiently listen to your concerns and answer your questions. They will teach you the best ways to touch your baby if you can't hold him. If your baby can be held, they will help you maneuver around any IVs or other medical devices that may be attached to him. They will help you learn to bathe and diaper your baby. If your baby is unable to breast-feed, the nurses will likely encourage you to pump your breast milk so they can feed it to him through a feeding tube as soon as he's able to eat. These things may sound trivial but in fact they are essential and will convince you that you are an important part of your baby's care.

Bonding Under Difficult Circumstances

If your newborn must spend some time in the NICU, you may wonder how—or even if—you can bond with him. As we stated earlier, we don't believe that bonding consists of one magic moment. Rather, it is an experience that takes place over time.

Spending time with your baby, even if he's confined to a NICU, is very important for both of you. Nevertheless, the NICU can be a very intimidating place—the unfamiliar sounds, machines, and smells, the knowledge that the babies in this special nursery are often very sick, the physical and emotional stress you're already feeling because of your Cesarean. It all adds up to a situation that can quickly become overwhelming. Remember that the nurses and physicians who are taking care of your baby care about you, too. When Dana's son was confined to the NICU for the first month of his life, the nurses encouraged her to read to him, to touch him, to sing to him, to decorate his tiny crib with photos, and to help with his care as much as possible. Mothers of sick newborns often report feelings of detachment, as if their baby belongs to the nurses and doctors rather than to them, but participating in your baby's basic care will help lessen those feelings.

How to Be Your Baby's Advocate When He's in the NICU

If you're in the midst of a health crisis with your newborn, you will find it difficult to remember to eat, let alone keep track of what your baby's caregivers are telling you about his health. "Parents tend to do a lot of head nodding because they don't want to seem ignorant," says Andy Spooner, MD, a spokesperson for the American Academy of Pediatrics. Some parents may also feel uncomfortable about asking too many questions about their child's health and medical treatment, because they don't want to irritate the doctors, fearing it may compromise the child's care. That's one thing you don't need to worry about, promises Dr. Spooner, since no pediatric physician is going to let his or her feelings about the family get in the way of the child's best interests. Here are a few tips that will help you be your child's best advocate:

- **Be assertive.** You have the right to ask questions about any treatments your child's physicians may recommend. Even if this is difficult for you, remember that the doctors want you to be informed about and understand your choices.

- **Write it down.** Keep a notebook with you at all times and write down questions and concerns you have for the doctors and nurses. Don't be shy about asking them to repeat or better explain information that you don't understand.

- **Get a second pair of ears.** Recruit a family member to take on the role as your second pair of ears during meetings with your child's health-care givers. Another person may hear things that you don't.

- **Get the help you need.** Ask to meet with the hospital's social worker. This person will help coordinate whatever follow-up care is required for your child after he's released from the hospital. A social worker can also help you find everything from support groups to financial aid.

CHAPTER 5

Breast-feeding: How to Guarantee Success

et's get the painful truth out of the way first: breast-feeding can be very challenging, even following the most uncomplicated delivery. When you're physically drained, in a fair amount of pain, and expected to snuggle with your newborn and be his sole source of nutrition, all we can say is—*Help!* While the last thing you are up for is more discomfort, know that sore nipples and swollen breasts will gradually disappear, just like the pain from your incision will decrease over time.

The first thing that surprises many first-time nursing moms is that breast-feeding, even though it's "natural," isn't always easy to get the hang of. And no matter how dedicated you are to breast-feeding, there will be times when you think it would be soooo much simpler to reach for a bottle of formula. But know that with a lot of determination and helpful advice, you will increase your chances of success and be able to enjoy one of the most fulfilling experiences you will have as a new mom. And once you get the hang of it, it can be more efficient and carefree than preparing bottle after bottle! We've also heard dozens of women say that breast-feeding after their Cesarean helped assuage some of the negative feelings they had about the surgical birth.

Our goal here is to help you get over some common obstacles, if breast-feeding is something you want to do. If all new moms were armed with just a few pieces of basic information *and* they asked for extra help while they were still in the hospital, the rate of breast-feeding would be much higher than it currently is. Although the American Academy of Pediatrics (AAP) recommends that babies drink breast milk *exclusively* for the first six months of life, only 64 percent of women even try to nurse. At six months, only 29 percent of moms are still breast-feeding; at one year, that number drops to 16 percent.

Six Reasons to Commit

Here's one undisputed fact: breast milk is the ideal food for newborn babies. And while we really don't want to sound preachy (we know that can be a total turn-off for women who are on the fence about breast-feeding), there are a few facts that might help you commit. (1) Dozens of studies have proven that breast-fed infants are healthier than formula-fed babies, especially during the first year of life. That's because invaluable immunities are passed to your infant through your milk, protecting him from colds and other respiratory infections, ear infections, and gastrointestinal illnesses. (2) Other studies have suggested that breast-fed babies have a lower risk of childhood obesity, and of developing serious diseases such as diabetes and even some forms of cancer. (3) Some of the most recent research suggests that breast-fed babies have IQs that are an average of seven to ten points higher than babies who are fed formula. (4) You benefit too. Women who breast-feed for six to twenty-four months cumulatively during their reproductive years may reduce their risk of breast cancer by 11–25 percent. (5) Nursing stimulates the contractions that will help your uterus heal and rebound to its previous size sooner than if you don't breast-feed. (6) Nursing also burns tons of calories, which may help you get back to your prepregnancy weight more quickly!

Those six reasons are very convincing—until you actually try to sit and hold your newborn to your breast. In the days and weeks following surgery, just sitting up can be painful enough, forget trying to hold a squirming, screaming baby in your arms. Between us, we have experienced nearly every bump in the road to breast-feeding, from breast infections to pumping problems to a preemie baby who was unable to latch on at first. Here are ten tips that we hope will make the experience easier for *you*.

#1. Tell everyone you plan to nurse.

As soon as you learn you'll be having a c-section, whether it's weeks or minutes before the surgery, make it known to your partner, your physician, the nurses, and even your parents, that you plan to breast-feed and want to nurse your baby as soon as possible following delivery. It's likely that your arms will be restrained until your OB has finished stitching up your uterus and abdomen, but with the help of your spouse and a nurse, you should still be able to try within the first few minutes of birth, a time when your baby is likely to be alert.

After your vital signs have been taken, and the baby has undergone the APGAR test, request that baby be handed over to you (or, more likely, to your partner since you won't be able to actually hold him). Depending on your IV setup, you may be able to roll to one side and have your partner prop the baby on a pillow so your baby can reach your breast. Or you may need someone to hold the baby on your chest for you. Don't be embarrassed—the medical professionals who are attending to you have seen it all before and should be willing to help however they can. Plus, you should take advantage of this time when you are painfree, thanks to the anesthesia, and can focus completely on loving your new baby. When one study compared twenty infants who were born via Cesarean and were allowed to suckle early after delivery with twenty who suckled later and were given supplementary food in the meantime, researchers found that the babies in the "early" category were more likely to get the hang of nursing.

If your baby is so drowsy that he won't even try to nurse, snuggle him to your breast anyway. The skin-to-skin contact will soothe him and he'll be comforted by your warmth and the familiar sound of your heartbeat. The contact will also stimulate your milk-making hormones.

If you are ultimately separated from your baby, either because you had general anesthesia and are in the recovery room without him, or because he had to be taken to the newborn nursery for observation or to undergo medical procedures, you *will* be able to breast-feed. You'll just require an extra dose of determination and maybe a few consultations with a lactation nurse. The idea that a baby who doesn't nurse within the first hours of birth will never "get it" is simply not true. One of us wasn't able to nurse her firstborn until he was three weeks old because he was confined to a NICU. It took some patience and a whole lot of pumping (see #7: Prepare to Pump) but he finally got the hang of it and ultimately nursed until he was eighteen months old.

#2. Be informed—and ask for help.

The emotional and physical stress of surgery, the anesthesia, post-operative pain medicine, and even gas pains may affect your initial attempts to nurse. If you went through several hours of labor before your c-section, you may be exhausted. If you had general anesthesia it will likely be several hours before you are even able to hold your baby, let alone try to breast-feed. Babies who are born via c-section are often more lethargic and therefore less willing to nurse than babies who are born vaginally. Does that sound like a bunch of bad news? Well, simply being aware of these factors may help you get through the early challenges.

If your hospital doesn't have a staff nursing consultant, you may want to schedule at least one appointment with one of these breast-feeding experts anyway. Some insurance companies will cover the cost of hospital and home visits with a private lactation consultant (your obstetrician or the nursing staff will be able to refer you to one), especially if the baby is premature or has other medical issues. If yours won't foot the bill, the investment is still worthwhile—and will probably cost you less than a month's worth of formula! Most hospitals also have certified lactation nurses on staff, so ask that one pay you a visit as soon as possible. Lactation nurses are well versed in the difficulties facing moms who are recovering from Cesarean surgery and they have both the experience and the patience to help you get through these initial challenges. They are also more objective than partners and parents and sometimes it's comforting to be able to voice your frustrations and fears to someone and not have to worry about being judged.

#3. Request the right roommate—your baby.

Unless either you or your baby experiences a medical difficulty, there is virtually no reason that he can't room with you. Some hospitals have a policy that babies who are born via Cesarean must be observed in the nursery for twenty-four hours, but if your baby is healthy, ask that the policy be waived; the on-call pediatrician should accommodate your request.

One reason having your baby in your room is so important is that it gives you a chance to learn his hunger cues. Most babies will root (a reflex that makes them open their mouth and move their head from side to side in search of mom's breast), make sucking noises, and pedal their legs as they start to get hungry. Crying is the last resort, and a sign that no one has responded to his earlier requests for food. But if your baby is in the newborn nursery, crying may be the *first* sign of hunger that the nurses notice, so by the time someone delivers baby to you, he's a screaming ball of fire. He's mad, you're tense, and getting him to latch on may be next to impossible (see #5: Learn What Makes a Good Latch). When he's next to you, though, and you can see or hear those initial signals, and have plenty of time to get comfortable, relax, and get him latched on before he's upset.

By having your baby with you, you are also more aware of his sleeping and waking cycles, which allows you to try to nurse during the times when he is most alert. It is also less likely that your newborn will be given bottles of formula or a pacifier if he is by your side. If for any reason, however, your baby is given a bottle in the nursery, breast-feeding is not doomed. He may seem confused, but if you offer him your breast often enough he should learn to prefer you.

If you have trouble convincing the hospital staff to let your baby room with you because you won't have a partner or friend with you at all times, ask that a student nurse be assigned to you. The majority of hospitals these days are teaching hospitals that have a number of students doing part of their training on-site. Student nurses are generally very enthusiastic and helpful. If you don't have family or friends who can help you with the baby while you're still in the hospital, a student nurse could be a great asset.

#4. Get comfortable and take your pain meds.

A basic fundamental of breast-feeding is your comfort. While women around the world have always breast-fed babies during some truly stressful times, such as war or famine, stress and fatigue can interfere with the hormones that make milk. One essential thing you can during the first few days following your surgery to promote breast-feeding is to take your pain medication. Many moms are so concerned that the drugs will be passed to their baby through their breast milk that they are reluctant to take any medicine (see the box, "Drugs in Breast Milk: What You Need to Know"). Don't be a martyr! Trace amounts of some medications do pass into the colostrum, the initial thin yellowish fluid that is rich in antibodies, protein, vitamins, and minerals and is so protective and nourishing to newborns that it's often called "liquid gold." The actual milk, which your baby will consume in much greater volume, won't arrive for three to six days. By that point you shouldn't need the strong narcotic drugs.

You may even ask your physician if you can receive intravenous pain medication for the first few days following surgery. One Japanese study found that women who had their epidurals left in place (and received analgesic pain relief intravenously) for three days following Cesarean surgery, breast-fed their babies more often and that the babies gained more weight than women who took oral pain medication. Stress—and anyone who's had one knows that a Cesarean can be *very* stressful—reduces production of the hormones oxytocin and prolactin, which are needed to produce breast milk, so be sure to manage your pain. When you're pain free you can relax more. Relaxation is key to breast-feeding because it ensures that your "milk ejection reflex" (also called "let down") kicks in.

Since you've had abdominal surgery, some things that you take for granted—getting up out of a chair or bed, walking up stairs, bending over to tie your shoes—may be quite challenging for the next couple of weeks. It won't take you *nearly* that long to find a breast-feeding position that suits both you and

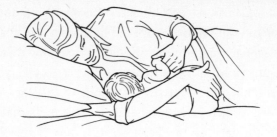

Figure 2. Nursing in the side-lying position.

your baby, but at first you'll probably have the best luck with three positions: lying down on one side, sitting up with a pillow on your lap so baby rests on top, and sitting up with baby in the clutch or "football" hold.

1. **Side-lying (Figure 2).** On the first day and maybe even for the first several weeks, lying down will be one of the more comfortable positions for you to nurse. (If your gas pains make it too uncomfortable to lie down, see position 2 below.) This will also be the position you come to rely on for middle-of-the-night feedings. If you're still in the hospital, make sure you bed is in the flat position. Ask your partner to gently wedge a pillow behind your back for support. Bend your knees and place another pillow between them for extra support; this also takes strain off your aching abdominal muscles. Ask your partner or a nurse to place your baby on his side, facing you, so you are chest to chest. His head should rest on your arm, or on a rolled-up towel or blanket. Make sure his mouth is at the same level as your breast to make it easy for him to latch on properly. Once baby has nursed from one breast, turn over and offer him the other breast.

2. **The clutch or "football" hold (Figure 3).** Sit in a comfortable armchair or sit up in bed. Place one or two pillows at

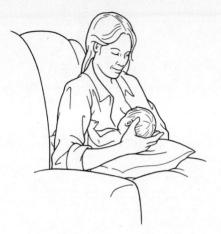

Figure 3. The clutch or football hold.

your side (on the side you will nurse from first), or wedge one between you and the side of the chair. Rest your baby on the pillow so his head is at breast level. Cradle the back of his head and neck between your thumb and forefinger, so that the palm of your hand is under his shoulders. His feet should be pointing behind you, his legs tucked under your armpit. His body should be bent at the hips with his bottom resting on the pillow or on your forearm. Bring his head to your breast and make sure he has latched on properly. Switch pillows and baby to the opposite side and repeat.

3. **The pillow prop (Figure 4).** Sitting up in bed or in a chair, place a pillow on your lap. If you have a special breast-feeding pillow that wraps partway around your waist, even better. Prop another pillow under the arm that's on the side you will nurse from first. Now place your baby on top of the pillow so he's not resting directly on your incision. Cradle him so his head rests in the crook of your elbow, his body rests on your forearm, and your hand cups his bottom. Tuck his

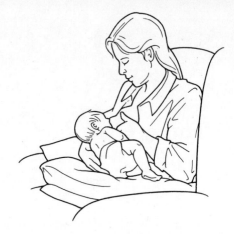

Figure 4. The pillow prop.

arm under yours. He should be tummy-to-tummy and face-to-breast with you. Make sure his back isn't arched backward and then bring him up and in toward your breast rather than leaning down to meet him (this will strain your back and may cause him to pull unnecessarily on your nipple).

During the coming months, you will discover a dozen different ways to hold your baby while you nurse and probably settle on one or two favorites. You'll also be surprised at the things you'll find yourself doing with a baby attached to your breast—one of us once had a pedicure while breast-feeding!—and before you know it, you'll forget these early challenges.

Be willing to try different nursing positions

"My incision ached and none of the positions I'd used with my first two babies were comfortable. It wasn't until a friend suggested I try resting my daughter on a horseshoe-shaped pillow that I found a position that worked. I wrapped the pillow around me and laid Hadley on top. That way she wasn't resting right on my tummy and it also relieved back pressure because I didn't have to hunch over. Even though I breast-fed my other two kids, what worked following my vaginal births didn't work with the Cesarean delivery. If I hadn't tried something new, those first few weeks would have been really miserable."

—Cheryl, mother of three, one Cesarean in 2002

#5. Learn what makes a good latch.

A proper "latch," the term used to describe the way a baby takes hold of the breast, is essential. Unfortunately, getting a newborn to latch the correct way can take some trial and error. The biggest mistake that new moms make with the latch is letting baby nurse only the tip of the nipple. Not only is this unbelievably painful (the last thing you need right now!), but it also prevents your baby from fully stimulating the breasts' milk sinuses, meaning he will have trouble getting enough milk.

To avoid an improper latch, cup your breast with one hand (you will have to experiment to see which hand you're more comfortable using) and use your thumb and index finger to form a "C" around your nipple and areola, the dark brown area of skin that surrounds your nipple.

Now tickle your baby's lips with your nipple until he turns his head toward you and opens his mouth. (If he turns his head away, use your finger to stroke his cheek that is closest to your breast. The "rooting" reflex will make him turn toward your breast.) As he opens his mouth, holding your hand behind his head, pull him toward you rather than leaning down to him, which will strain your back. Once he starts to suckle, check to make sure his lips are flanged out, covering the nipple and at least a half-inch of the areola. In order for him to stimulate the milk sinuses, he must put pressure on the area around the nipple and not just suck on the nipple itself.

He should be so close to you that the tip of his nose touches your breast. Watch and listen for a rhythmic sucking pattern; if baby is chomping or biting in a frantic way, break the suction by sliding your finger between his mouth and your breast and start again. If you're still concerned that he's not latching on correctly, pull down his lower lip while he's nursing. You should be able to see his tongue between his lower lip and your breast. If you can't see his tongue, he's probably sucking on it as well as your nipple. Break the suction as described above and start again.

#6. Master the relaxation response.

For the first few days after your surgery, the discomfort you feel may make you doubt your ability to nurse. However, this minirelaxation exercise, courtesy of Alice Domar, PhD, a renowned mind/body expert, will help distract you from the pain so you can shift into a mind-set that will help you succeed.

- Sit quietly in a comfortable position. If possible, have your partner or someone else hold the baby while you do the next two steps.
- Close your eyes.
- Slowly count backward from ten to zero taking deep abdominal breaths while you count. (Breathing deeply will also help cleanse your lungs of residual anesthesia and reduce risk for postoperative respiratory difficulties, Domar says.) If the deep breaths are painful, try clutching a pillow to help support your tummy.
- Now position your baby to nurse.

If possible, practice the relaxation exercise several times throughout the day.

When you feel pain, or if your baby won't latch on, try this breathing exercise. You'll feel positively flooded by calm, promises Domar.

#7. Prepare to pump.

Babies who are born prematurely, or who must be hospitalized for any length of time following birth, are often unable to nurse. If your baby cannot start breast-feeding during the first twelve to twenty-four hours following birth, the best way to establish the milk supply that will be necessary to feed him when he *is* able to nurse is to pump or "express" milk.

Pumping early and often will also prevent the potentially painful engorgement that can occur when breast milk comes in. Every hospital has breast pumps available to patients who need them, and if it looks like breast-feeding will be delayed, you should request that one be brought to your room as soon as possible. In order to establish the milk supply necessary to nourish your newborn, you will need to pump as often as your baby would if he were able to nurse, typically about every two hours.

The very thought of pumping milk from their breasts makes some women a little squeamish (can you say "Moo?"), but it's not as awkward or uncomfortable as you may imagine. In fact, once you get the hang of it, it's pretty simple. And if you get into the habit of pumping early, you will have more freedom (and maybe more sleep!) later because your spouse or a babysitter will be able to feed your baby expressed breast milk from a bottle. Breast milk can be frozen for up to six months so don't worry that your efforts will be wasted. (For tips on storing breast milk, see "Breast-feeding FAQs.")

The breast pumps used in hospitals are very efficient: with a hospital-grade "double" automatic-cycling pump, you can express both breasts simultaneously and empty your breasts in about ten minutes. During the first week, try to pump between eight to ten times a day. Since rest is vital both for your recovery and for making milk, don't worry about pumping throughout the night; unless your breasts are very full and leaking, you should be able to get away with pumping just once in the middle of the night. By the second week, you can cut back to about five to eight sessions a day, pumping every two to three hours during the daytime hours. To help you keep track of how often you're pumping, try to schedule your first session on the hour, say 7 a.m. or 8 a.m. The next session would then start at 10 a.m. or 11 a.m.

Hospital-grade pumps are available to rent. If your baby must remain in the hospital after you are discharged, we highly recommend that you rent a pump to keep at home. The hospital staff can help you arrange for a rental, though large pharmacies such as CVS and Walgreens typically stock them. Your insurance company may cover the cost of the rental, which averages about $50 per month, so it's worth checking into. Be sure to have your baby's pediatrician, or the physician who is caring for your baby in the hospital, write a prescription for a breast pump *in the baby's name* before you arrange to rent the pump. If the prescription is in mom's name, it's harder to get reimbursement. We know of one insurance company that gives *every* new mom a $200 breast pump before she checks out of the hospital. Since insurance companies are notoriously frugal, we can only assume that executives at this company are convinced that the health-protecting benefits of breast-feeding for both mom and baby will ultimately save them money in claims down the road. It might be worth asking your insurance provider if they are willing to cover the cost, or part of the cost, for a pump.

If you are committed to breast-feeding but know that you will be returning to work during the first few months following your baby's birth, you might also consider buying a pump. Several companies, including Medela, Ameda, Bailey Medical Engineering, and Whittlestone, manufacture portable electric double-pumps that are nearly as efficient as the hospital pumps and they cost between $120 and $350. Battery-operated and handheld "bicycle horn" pumps are very inexpensive but are not adequate to use for frequent pumping.

Don't be afraid of the pump

"My son was confined to the neonatal intensive care unit for almost the first month of his life. He was so sick that he couldn't nurse until he was almost three weeks old, but every day, throughout the day, I pumped breast milk for the nurses to give him through a feeding tube. For much of his time in the NICU I felt so helpless—I couldn't hold him, change his diapers or bathe him—so at least by pumping I felt like I was doing something positive for him. Once he was finally healthy, he started nursing and I ultimately breast-fed him until he was eighteen months old."

—Dana, mother of three, Cesareans in 1997, 1999, 2004

#8. Set up a nursing nest at home.

Getting comfortable goes beyond finding the best way to hold your baby while you nurse. Remember that "comfort is key." In the beginning you may be nursing for up to forty-five minutes at a time, so setting up a little nursing sanctuary for yourself will help you settle into the nursing routine. The way you furnish your nest is up to you, of course, but some items that we found helpful included:

- A rocking or gliding chair with a comfy cushion. This is an expense, but it is well worth it. If you can splurge on an ottoman or footstool, all the better. Keeping your feet raised while you nurse will take pressure off your incision and your back, and it's more comfortable to nurse if your feet are elevated slightly.

- A few pillows to help you prop your baby on your lap or to help you sit comfortably.
- A basket that has a few nutritious snacks in it, such as dried fruit, nuts, or some granola bars.
- A water bottle to help you stay hydrated throughout the day. Drink to satisfy your thirst, which will probably be about 48–64 ounces (that's six to eight 8-ounce glasses) but pay attention to your body's signals. If your urine is dark, that means it's very concentrated and you need more fluids. On the other hand, if you are feeling bloated, you may be drinking too much, which can actually decrease your milk production.
- Hand wipes so you can clean your hands before breast-feeding.
- A cordless phone, if you don't find talking on the phone too distracting.
- A paperback book or magazine.
- A radio or remote control so you can listen to music or watch television if you prefer.

#9. Let your baby set his own schedule

Nursing babies feed often. So often, in fact, that you might feel like all you're doing during the first few weeks of your baby's life is changing his diapers and unhooking your nursing bra. It won't be this way forever or even for very long, we promise. "Watch your baby and not the clock," is the advice lactation nurses give. During the first few weeks of life, a newborn may suck for five minutes, or forty-five minutes. How long and how frequently your baby nurses depends on him, though most newborns feed every two hours or sometimes more often for the first month or two.

The more frequently you nurse, the higher the fat and calorie content of your milk, making it better for your baby. The breast makes milk fastest when it's empty so the more often you nurse the greater your milk supply. A study that looked at the frequency of suckling—a study tellingly titled, "The Frequency of Sucking: A neglected but essential ingredient of breast-feeding"—suggests that the frequency of feeding decreases nipple pain and breast tenderness, and noticeably increases milk output and infant weight gain. The bottom line is that if you "nurse early and nurse often," you will make great strides toward breast-feeding success.

#10. Be aware of potential pitfalls.

Sometimes, despite your best efforts, difficulties do arise during the initial days of breast-feeding. It will be helpful if you're aware of the most common ones—and know how to deal with them.

- **Sore nipples or painful nursing.** Your nipples will toughen up, but during these early days, especially if your baby has trouble with latching on, they may be sore. The first way to combat sore nipples to is perfect the latch (see tip #5). All skin, including the skin on your breasts, heals more quickly if it's exposed to air. Breast milk actually contains healing properties that you can easily take advantage of. When your baby has finished nursing, rub the milk that's left behind into your breast. Then allow the skin to air dry before putting your bra back on. Avoid using plastic-lined breast pads or shields since they can trap moisture.

- **Engorgement.** The best way to relieve engorgement—which can occur right after your milk comes in, or later if you go several hours without nursing—is to nurse often. Taking a warm shower or bath, or placing warm compresses on your breasts may also relieve the pain of engorgement.

- **Breast tenderness from plugged milk ducts.** If one area of your breast suddenly becomes sore, or if you feel a lump in your breast, the most likely cause is a plugged milk duct. Milk ducts can become plugged if your baby misses a feeding (it's quite normal for this to happen when a baby begins sleeping through the night and mom must go for several hours between feedings), but wearing a bra that is too tight or has underwires that pinch can also cause this problem. The best way to heal a plugged duct is to apply heat to the breast—either a heating pad or a wet compress works well, to nurse your baby often *from the sore side*, and to make sure that your bra isn't too constricting. It's also important to rest as much as possible when you have plugged ducts.

- **Mastitis.** A breast infection, also known as mastitis, can make you feel like you have the flu. You will probably have a fever and feel generally run-down. At first, you should treat a breast infection the same way you would a plugged duct: frequent nursing, the application of heat, and rest. But if your fever lasts for more than twenty-four hours, you should call your doctor because you may need an antibiotic to combat the infection. A breast infection can quickly become systemic and may even require hospitalization and intravenous antibiotics, so it is imperative that you seek treatment for a suspected infection as soon as possible.

- **Yeast infection of the breast, also called thrush.** If your breasts become tender and painful and you notice the skin around your nipple is pink and flaky, you may have a fungal infection called thrush. Your baby may also come down with the same infection in his mouth (marked by white spots), and on his bottom, in the form of diaper rash that just won't heal. Thrush thrives in warm, moist environments. Your pediatrician will prescribe a topical solution for your baby and probably for you as well. There is no reason to stop nursing because of thrush and it should heal within a couple of weeks.

Breast-feeding FAQs

Q. **Do I need to prepare my breasts for breast-feeding?**

A. Probably not. The hormones of pregnancy do a great job of preparing breasts for their starring role. If your nipples are very sensitive, however, you might try going braless for the last few weeks of your pregnancy. If that's uncomfortable, wear a nursing bra with the flaps down. The light rubbing against your clothing will help "condition" your nipples. You should also avoid using soap on your nipples because it can by drying.

Q. **When does breast milk come in?**

A. Usually within five days after your baby's birth. Until the milk appears, though, your baby is getting colostrum, a thick, yellowish premilk that is rich in protein and immunities. You'll know when your milk comes in because your breasts will suddenly feel very full and firm, and may be quite hard and sore at first.

Q. **How do I know if my baby is getting enough milk?**

A. A baby who is getting enough breast milk has at least six very wet diapers every day plus two seedy stools. His stools should change during the first few weeks, too. They start out sticky and black and change from green to brown to mustard yellow after a month or so. If your baby seems content, if he sucks vigorously and swallows, he is probably getting enough milk. At his two-week checkup he should be back to his birth weight. If you're worried that your baby isn't gaining enough, call your pediatrician's office and ask to schedule a "weight check."

Q. If I have to pump, how do I safely store my expressed breast milk?

A. Store breast milk in clear plastic or glass bottles, or specially designed plastic freezer bags that secure with twist ties or mini plastic clips. Any of these storage containers can go into the freezer. The type of refrigerator/freezer you have determines the length of time breast milk can be safely stored (be sure to date each container).

In a refrigerator:
- At 32°F-39°F, 8 days
- At 59°F-60°F, 24 hours
- At 66°F-71.6°F, 10 hours
- At 79°F, 4–8 hours

In a freezer:
- In the freezer compartment inside a refrigerator (such as those found in hotel "minibars"), 2 weeks
- In the freezer of a refrigerator/freezer (either side-by-side or top-bottom models), 3 or 4 months
- In a "deep freeze," freezer where the temperature is 0°F, 6 months

Q. Can breast-feeding prevent pregnancy?

A. One of us has a sibling who is 360 days younger than she is. Without getting too personal, let's just say her mom relied on breast-feeding for contraception and it didn't work. She ended up with a set of "Irish twins." Still, frequent nursing *can* suppress ovulation, making it less likely that you're menstruating or ovulating regularly. Lactation consultants say there are three criteria for preventing pregnancy while breast-feeding, a method of contraception known as the lactation amenorrhea method (LAM). First, your baby must be younger than six months of age. Second, the baby must nurse exclusively (that means no supplemental bottles or pacifiers). And third, your period must not have resumed. Once just one of those criteria can't be met you will need a backup method, and LAM is only 98 percent effective so there are no guarantees! If you do not want to be pregnant, do not use breast-feeding as birth control.

You should talk with your physician about other options. The American College of Obstetricians and Gynecologists currently recommends that women who are breast-feeding use barrier methods of contraception (e.g., condoms, spermicide, diaphragm, copper IUD) rather than hormones. According to ACOG, hormones (birth control pills, injections such as Depo-Provera, implants, and patches) pose a "theoretical" risk to nursing infants and are generally not recommended to nursing moms. Even the progestin-only options (called the "mini pill") aren't recommended during the early days of breast-feeding because they can affect milk production, and because the hormones are passed to the infant and some experts worry that a baby could have trouble metabolizing the drug. Once your baby is several weeks old, or if you are supplementing with formula, your physician may okay the mini pill.

Q. Should I be eating or drinking anything special while I breast-feed?

A. You need about 500 calories more than normal per day. If average intake for you is 2,000–2,200 calories, then you'll bump it up to about 2,500–2,700. As for what to eat, now is an ideal time to start eating nutritiously (if you haven't done so in the past) because not only will you pass the nutrients from your own healthy diet on to your baby through your breast milk, but you'll also lose your pregnancy weight more quickly if you cut out some of the sugar and fat that are so prevalent in the

American diet. Use the U.S. Department of Agriculture's Food Guide Pyramid as a starting point (http://www.usda.gov/cnpp/pyrabklt.pdf). Beyond that:

- **Keep an eye on your calcium intake.** Aim for 1,000 milligrams a day to keep your bones healthy. Rich sources of calcium include skim milk, calcium-fortified orange juice, yogurt, canned salmon and sardines, kale and other greens, tofu, and dried beans.

- **Fulfill your daily folate requirement.** Folate (folic acid) is a vitamin that was essential during pregnancy (to help prevent certain birth defects, such as spina bifida) but you need it when you're breast-feeding, too. The Food and Drug Administration (FDA) recommends that nursing women get 400 micrograms daily. You can get folic acid from a prenatal vitamin/mineral supplement, or from enriched grains (e.g., some breakfast cereals and breads and pastas) or from spinach, citrus fruits, cauliflower, broccoli, lentils, and legumes.

- **Don't forget the vitamin D.** Vitamin D helps your body absorb calcium, which is essential for healthy bones. The two best ways to get it are from fifteen minutes of direct sunlight a day (wearing sunscreen, of course), or from drinking enriched milk. If you don't do either, be sure to get your recommended daily allowance of Vitamin D (5 mcg) from a supplement.

- **Docosahexanenoic acid is a must-do.** Of the dozens of known "ingredients" found in human breast milk, one of the most important is docosahexaenoic acid (DHA), a long-chain polyunsaturated fatty acid. It promotes both neurological and visual development. In fact, it is among the most important structures in the human brain. Your baby will get plenty of DHA through your breast milk, but you need to boost your own since it takes many months for your body to get back to its normal DHA levels after pregnancy. During these sleep-deprived nights, the more you can do to boost your mental acuity, the better! Foods such as fish (see below for warnings about certain types of fish), red meat, and eggs are good sources of DHA.

Q: Are there any foods I should avoid?

A: This is a tough one. Some babies are more sensitive to what their mothers have eaten than others. You've probably heard that certain foods, like cruciferous vegetables (e.g., broccoli, cauliflower) cause gas, but this isn't always the case. So rather than just cut out every potentially gas-causing food from your diet, or the ones like garlic and peppers that you think might distress your baby, experiment. Keep a food diary and if two to twelve hours after eating a certain food, your baby is fussy, then cut it out of your diet for a while. Corn, soy milk, wheat, eggs, peanuts, and shellfish are the foods that most commonly upset a baby's tummy.

And there are some modifications that all nursing moms want to make to their diet. You want to limit your intake of fish that contain high levels of mercury, including swordfish and shark. Up to 12 ounces of canned fish, shellfish and other smaller ocean fish can be consumed per week. If you are losing significant amounts of weight (more than two pounds a week), after six weeks postpartum, you could pass mercury to your baby through breast milk since the mercury is stored in fat tissue. (For more info, go to the U.S. Environmental Protection Agency's Web Site at www.epa.gov.)

Q: I've had breast augmentation or reduction surgery. Can I still breast-feed?

A: It depends on how the procedure was done. If you've had the surgery recently, then chances are the implants were inserted through an incision near the armpits, under the breast tissue, or under the chest muscle, which shouldn't interfere with breast-feeding.

If you've had surgery in which the nipple was removed to place the implant and then reattached, you will probably not be able to breast-feed because this procedure disrupts so many nerves in the breast that let down is impaired.

Women who've had reduction surgery often have more difficulty with breast-feeding, but it's not impossible for them, either. If the nipple is left partially attached during the procedure, and then reattached once the unwanted breast tissue has been removed, it is more likely that you'll be able to breast-feed.

In either case, be sure to you let your pediatrician know you've had surgery so she can keep a close watch on your baby's weight gain. Some women who have had breast surgery need to supplement with formula. And if you are considering breast surgery but plan to breast-feed in the future, be sure to talk with your surgeon about using a technique that will make breast-feeding possible.

Drugs and Breast Milk: What You Need to Know

You may be surprised by the number of medications you're prescribed following Cesarean surgery. Typically, you're given pain medication—which may contain a narcotic such as codeine—an antibiotic, and a stool-softener. Depending on the circumstances of your delivery, you may also be given medication for high blood pressure. In rare situations, women are prescribed antianxiety or antidepressant drugs.

Even if all you take is Tylenol, you may be concerned that the medication will have a negative effect on your baby. In fact, according to the AAP, one of the reasons that many women stop nursing is that they receive their physician's advice to do so because of concerns about medication tainting breast milk. However, *in most cases*, the amounts of drugs frequently prescribed postpartum that pass through breast milk are so small that the baby will not be harmed.

There are some drugs, however, whose effects are considered "unknown but of concern." To protect your newborn, be sure to ask your pediatrician to reference the article "The Transfer of Drugs and Other Chemicals into Human Milk," which was published in *Pediatrics* in September 2001 (you can also read the list online at http://www.aap.org/policy/0063.html). It lists hundreds of drugs and their potential effects on a nursing baby.

The AAP also recommends that before using any medication, a breast-feeding mother should always choose the safest option (e.g., acetaminophen for pain rather than aspirin), and that a mom can minimize baby's drug exposure by taking the medication just after breast-feeding or just before the infant is due to have a long nap.

Finally, it goes without saying (but we'll say it anyway) that illegal drugs, such as amphetamines, cocaine, heroin, phencyclidine, and marijuana are extremely dangerous to your nursing newborn.

CHAPTER 6

Healing at Home

We're going to let you in on a little secret. Pregnancy isn't really three trimesters. It's four! Truly, if our culture considered the postpartum recovery period part of pregnancy, we suspect fewer women would feel so overwhelmed by new motherhood. In other parts of the world, new mothers are practically worshipped during the first few weeks after giving birth. In India, for example, new mothers are encouraged to stay home and be pampered for twenty-two days after giving birth. In Holland, new mothers are routinely treated to live-in help (in the form of a midwife) for eight days postpartum. In the United Kingdom, new moms are visited at home six or seven times by a midwife during the first two weeks postpartum. That's standard for a vaginal delivery!

In the United States, we are lucky if we get a single home visit from a nurse, and even that is usually offered only to women who have delivered by Cesarean. Here, many women feel compelled to get on with their lives as soon as they can after childbirth. We urge you to consider the first six weeks—or more, if possible—as a time when you should be waited on and even exalted. Don't feel compelled to answer the phone every time it rings or entertain every visitor who stops by "just for a minute." (Posting a sign that says "Baby is sleeping" on your front door should cut back on the intrusions.)

We know we don't have to tell you, but women who deliver

by Cesarean have some special concerns during the postpartum period. For starters, you are much more fatigued than women who have vaginal births. You can expect to feel pretty wiped out for at least the next couple of weeks. It's important for every new mom to conserve her energy, but it's vital for women who are recovering from a c-section. Your physician gave you specific instructions about what you should and should not do during the first six weeks, and even though some of them—like not vacuuming—might seem silly, she gave them to you for a reason. Strenuous activity, including lifting anything heavier than your baby, could open your incision.

Focus on You

During the first few weeks postpartum, you need to take care of yourself so you can take care of your baby. Let your spouse, family, and friends do everything else. It can take between four to eight weeks for your incision to heal completely. So the less strenuous your activity is during these early days, the easier your recovery will be, and the sooner you'll be able to handle those sleepless nights with a smile. (Okay, maybe not quite a smile.)

At the top of the list of concerns for women who have c-sections is the risk of infection. Even with the many precautions physicians and nurses take to combat bacteria, both in the operating room and afterward, there is a still a risk of developing an infection at the incision site or in the vagina or uterus. And until the incision is completely healed, it can become infected. Signs of a wound infection include fever, foul-smelling vaginal discharge, elevated pulse, redness and heat around the incision, and drainage from the site.

If you experience painful urination, or if urination becomes more difficult as the days go by, there is a chance that bacteria were introduced into your urinary tract when the catheter was inserted prior to surgery, and now there's an infection inside. If vaginal bleeding increases about five to eight days following surgery, if you feel really fatigued, and if you have increasing abdom-

When to Call Your Physician

If you notice any of the following signs in the days between your release from the hospital and your six-week checkup, call your physician right away, even if it's in the middle of the night:

- Bleeding that requires you to change your sanitary pad every hour. (If you're bleeding so heavily that you fill *more* than one pad per hour, have someone drive you to the emergency room or call 911.)
- Large blood clots in your vaginal discharge (called lochia), which could be a sign of excessive bleeding or possible hemorrhage.
- Foul-smelling lochia, which can indicate infection.
- No lochia during the first two weeks postpartum.
- Pain in the incision area or below that worsens rather than gets better, or a swollen incision that is red and feels warm to the touch, which are signs of infection. (The pain around your incision should lessen with each passing day.)
- A fever higher than about 100°F, which may indicate infection.
- Pain or difficulty with urination, very dark urine, or very little urine coming out when you try to empty your bladder, which are signs of a urinary tract infection.
- Pain or tenderness in your lower legs, or pain when you flex your ankles, which are signs of a potential blood clot in the leg. Elevate your leg and call your physician as soon as possible.
- Sharp chest pain, which can indicate a blood clot in the lungs. Call your physician, but if you can't reach her immediately, have someone drive you to the emergency room or call 911.

inal pain, call your doctor right away because you may have a uterine infection. The earlier you catch any postpartum infection, the better the odds that it can be treated with oral antibiotics.

. . . .

Pay attention to your incision

"About a week after my Cesarean, I woke up with a fever and noticed that my incision was red and really sore. The surgical tapes were still on, but the incision was definitely oozing and I knew that wasn't a good sign. I called my physician and he put me on antibiotics right away. I'm glad I didn't ignore the signs of the infection because I know other people who've had staph infections that required them to be readmitted to the hospital for intravenous antibiotics. I felt better within forty-eight hours and healed just fine after that. I was worried that I'd have to stop breast-feeding but my doctor told me the antibiotics wouldn't hurt my daughter."

—Cheryl, mother of three, one Cesarean in 2002

. . . .

Is This Normal?

Even though you might have been anxious to get out of the hospital and home to start life with your newborn, the hospital had its pluses. Besides the 24-hour meal and housekeeping service, there was probably comfort in knowing that if you had any questions about what to expect following your Cesarean, all you had to do was ring that little buzzer next to your bed. Once you're home, you're basically on your own.

Here are the answers to a few questions that might cross your mind:

- *I feel faint. Does that mean I lost a lot of blood during my Cesarean? How long can I expect to feel this way?* During the first few days after a delivery, your body goes through many changes. For starters, the fluids levels—including the blood volume that helped sustain your baby during pregnancy—changes, and these shifts can make you feel dizzy. Hormones are also fluctuating, which can also contribute to feelings of lightheadedness. Drinking plenty of water should help.

Another possible reason for feeling faint is that after surgery, the blood vessels in your legs might not be constricting the way they usually do, so when you stand up and the blood rushes to your legs, you feel faint. Try to stand up slowly.

Some women find that pain medications make them feel lightheaded but once they stop taking the painkillers that side effect disappears. Finally, if you lost a lot of blood during the surgery, or are anemic, you may also experience feelings of lightheadedness during the first few postpartum days. Getting plenty of rest, eating nutritiously, and drinking extra fluids will help.

- *My OB told me not to lift anything heavier than my baby. Why?* Even though your physician used strong sutures to sew up the layers she had to cut through to deliver your baby, it's better to avoid straining the incision during the first few weeks postpartum. The risk that you could open the incision is small, but it is always a possibility. Anyway, your physician doesn't want you overextending yourself right now and if you are lifting heavy objects—baskets of laundry, bags of groceries, etc.—you're doing too much.

- *I'm sweating a lot. Is that normal?* If you're sweating because you have a fever, you need to call your physician because you may have developed an infection. Otherwise, it's probably just a sign that your body is getting rid of some of the excess fluids that accumulated during pregnancy. It shouldn't last more than a few days. You might have to sleep on a towel to soak up the sweat at night. To protect your mattress, slide a crib-sized waterproof pad under your sheet.

- *When can I take a bath? What about swimming?* Most women

are given the go-ahead to shower before they leave the hospital. One reason that your physician might have recommended showers at home is because it can be challenging to climb in and out of the tub. If you can do that safely, there's no reason to stay out of the bath. However, you should not take a very hot bath because prolonged exposure to the heat could cause your blood pressure to drop and make you faint. Do not use bubble bath or bath oils because they may irritate your incision and possibly increase the risk of infection (if you long for a soothing scent, try burning an aromatherapy candle while you soak). Don't scrub off the surgical tape that is helping to hold the incision closed; each piece should fall off naturally within about two weeks. And just to be on the safe side, you shouldn't swim until the incision is healed; the risk of infection isn't worth it.

- *When is it safe to have sex?* Once you've gone two weeks without bleeding, it is safe to have intercourse again. After that—well, it's up to you.

- *I have diarrhea. Is something wrong?* Probably not. Your first few bowel movements after surgery may be very loose if you were given any laxatives or stool softeners. However, if you have watery diarrhea that lasts more than a couple of days, let your physician know. Sometimes the antibiotics that are given during labor or postpartum can cause temporary problems in your digestive system.

- *My physician told me not to drive for ten to fourteen days. Why?* There are a couple of good reasons to leave your car in park. First, you have just had surgery and you are tired, so you might not be able to react quickly in an unexpected traffic situation. Second, if you're still on narcotic medication, your judgment and reaction time while you're behind the wheel are not 100 percent (plus, if you got into an accident, and were on medication, there's a good chance you'd be held liable). And finally, you're supposed to be home recovering from your Cesarean and taking care of your baby. You don't need to be out shopping or visiting; it's taxing for you and it exposes your newborn to a whole range of germs that he'd be better off without during the first few weeks of his life. Since your first post-op visit and your baby's first visit with the pediatrician are likely to be scheduled before you should be behind the wheel, arrange to have someone drive you to your appointments.

- *Is vacuuming really going to hurt me?* You do exert your abdominal muscles when you move the vacuum back and forth, so resist the urge to run it for a few days. Besides, a little dust and dirt never hurt anyone. If you're worried about what people might think if they come to visit and your house isn't in tip-top shape, well, let us remind you that you just had a baby—by Cesarean. If anything, when your mom, dad, spouse, next door neighbor, or friend ask if they can help, have them do things like vacuuming, emptying the dishwasher, and sprucing up the bathroom. After all, how many times in your life will you really have a good excuse for delegating chores like these?

Relieving Common Discomforts

Constipation, cramps, and mood swings. Oh, my! So this isn't quite what you expected from motherhood? Rest assured that all of these complaints are common, and they won't last long. In the meantime, here's what you can do to ease your pains:

- **Constipation (and hemorrhoids).** Bet you never thought you'd be so aware of what's going on down there. Constipation and hemorrhoids can often be avoided during pregnancy, but both are practically rites of passage for women who've delivered via Cesarean. The constipating effects of the postoperative pain medicine, plus the surgery itself, can be traumatic to the intestines and bowels. In fact, it's not unusual for a woman who's had a c-section to go three or four days postpartum without a bowel movement. Crossing that first hurdle—passing gas—which you did prior to your release from the hospital, means things in your intestines are starting to move again. And bowel function should follow soon.

Postpartum Rx: Increase your fluid intake (consider eight 8-ounce glasses of water the minimum), especially if you're breast-feeding, eat extra dietary fiber, and load up on fruits and vegetables, which help digestion. Certain juices, such as prune and apricot, will also help to get your bowels functioning again. It's a good idea to avoid constipating foods such as milk, ice cream, cheese, yogurt, bananas, and rice, and to increase your intake of fiber-rich foods such as bran muffins, shredded wheat cereals, oatmeal, and popcorn.

Short sitzbaths and/or cold packs also provide some relief. Ask your caregiver to recommend a nonprescription stool softener or mild laxative such as Milk of Magnesia, or a fiber additive like Citrucel, to help things loosen up. Using a gel or cream formula like Preparation H or a product with witch hazel, such as Tucks, will help ease the pain of hemorrhoids, which can last for several weeks postpartum. Doing Kegel exercises that focus on the muscles around the anus also speeds healing.

Natural Remedies for Common Complaints

If you feel like your Cesarean was all the medical intervention you want for the time being, you might consider using some natural remedies to treat what's ailing you. Here are a few time-tested remedies:

- **Tea bags to soothe sore nipples.** Soak a tea bag—it must be black tea which is rich in healing tannins, such as Lipton's—in warm water and place it over your nipples. Cover with a warm washcloth and sit for ten to fifteen minutes. Repeat every few hours as needed. Something in the tannin relieves the pain of sore, cracked nipples.

- **Chamomile tea to ease uterine cramps.** It's caffeine-free and seems to relieve the cramping that follows delivery. Nurse-midwives routinely give it to their patients while they're still in the recovery room and recommend that women drink it throughout the day. At home, keep it brewing: it's soothing and it's an ideal hydrating fluid when you want something other than plain water. If you are drinking a lot of tea, be aware that it can interfere with iron absorption. If you have low iron, you should not drink more than one or two cups of tea a day.

- **Potatoes and witch hazel to help heal hemorrhoids.** Yes, you read that correctly. Slice a potato and place it on your sore bottom for ten minutes, several times throughout the day. It's an old nurse-midwives' remedy that is still used today. If that's too "alternative" for you, try soaking a cotton pad in refrigerated witch hazel and placing it on your bottom for a few minutes.

- **Relax with lavender.** Place a silk lavender-and-flax-filled pillow over your eyes and feel the tension melt away (lavender is known for its sedative effects). You can also heat the pillow in a microwave and place it on your neck or back to soothe sore muscles. These pillows are available at health food stores.

- **Cramps and bleeding.** Your uterus has accomplished a difficult job—expanding to twenty-five times its normal size to accommodate a growing baby, and then being cut open. Now it must heal inside and out. The cramping is a sign that your uterus is contracting and shrinking back to its normal size. (It takes just six weeks for the uterus to return to its prepregnancy size.) Even though you had a c-section, you will still bleed vaginally, because the blood comes from the uterine wall and the newly exposed placental site. Bleeding also occurs when the scabs inside the uterus fall off before the site is fully healed.

Postpartum R$_x$: Breast-feed. Nursing stimulates the production of oxytocin, a hormone that stimulates the uterus to contract, which in turn helps speed its return to normal size. The contractions also reduce postpartum bleeding. If the pain is unbearable, your caregiver may recommend over-the-counter pain medication. For the bleeding, stock up on sanitary pads and be patient. Don't use tampons because they can introduce infection. The bleeding and discharge, called lochia, is usually red for the first week or so, then fades to pink, and then to yellow or white. Postpartum bleeding is often heavier than a menstrual period, but if you pass large clots of blood, soak more than one sanitary napkin per hour, if the bleeding increases rather than subsides, or if you notice a foul-smelling odor, be sure to call your physician. Any of these can be signs of hemorrhage, which may occur if there are still small pieces of the placenta attached to your uterus, or indicate an infection in your vagina or uterus.

- **Mood swings and fatigue.** You're a mom! You have a beautiful newborn! You can't believe how lucky you are! So why do you feel so blue? Because you had surgery, because you're exhausted, and because you're human. You're also in good company. It's completely normal for new moms to experience some sadness, tears, and irritability during the first few days and weeks postpartum. In fact, by some estimates, 80 percent of new moms experience "postpartum blues" for up to two weeks after delivery. Hormones are dipping and surging, you're sore, and motherhood may not be quite what you expected.

Postpartum R$_x$: Relax. And—it can't be said enough—you need sleep. Try to nap when your baby does, at least once during the day. If you can't do that, force yourself to go bed early. Accept all offers of help, and don't be shy about asking for it either. Make every effort to devote a little bit of time to yourself each day. Even taking a fifteen-minute walk or a bath may give you the recharge you need. If you're concerned that what you're feeling is more than sadness, for example, if your tears last more than two weeks or if you have feelings of guilt or anxiety, call your physician. True postpartum depression is relatively rare (about 10–20 percent of new moms have it and it's more widespread in women with a family history of depression), but if you're suffering from it, your caregiver can refer you to the help you need, which may include the temporary use of antidepressant medication. (For more information, see Chapter 7: Dealing with Mixed Emotions.)

Five Things You Can Do to Speed Your Recovery

It's one of those little ironies in life that the best preparation for having a newborn at home is having had one before. Short of that, nothing can really prepare you for the life-altering event that is a new baby. You may have had a certain vision of what your life would be like after you delivered your baby. And even if you knew before your due date that you were going to have a Cesarean birth, you still may have clung to some notions about what you could accomplish once you got home. All we can say is: let it go. The postpartum period is not dreadful, really; it can, however, be challenging. Here are five simple things you can do to make it go more smoothly:

1. **Lower your expectations.** What were your plans for mater-

nity leave? Were you going to clean closets, sort years' worth of photos into albums, organize your pantry, finally plan and plant a cutting garden? Who knows when you'll have a long stretch of time "off" again, so you might as well get as much done as possible, right? Wrong! Postpartum is not a synonym for vacation. You body has just gone through an extraordinary experience, you conceived and carried a baby, then you delivered that baby surgically, possibly following a tiring labor. The only thing you should do right now is rest and take care of your baby. All the things that you hoped to accomplish right now don't need to be done today or tomorrow. You don't have anything to prove to anyone (or to yourself), so take this time to snuggle with your baby and heal your body. Those photos will be there next year, and as long as you have a general idea of what's in your pantry, that's all that really matters.

2. **Accept all offers of help.** For starters, let your family and friends know that you really do need them. Make a list of all the errands and chores that need to be done. Write each chore on a small piece of paper and put the slips of paper in a basket or a paper bag. When anyone (and we mean anyone, even a neighbor you hardly know) calls or stops by and asks how they can help, reach into the basket and remove a slip of paper with a chore on it. In our experience, the people who offer really do want to help, even if it means coming by to drop off a meal, do a load of laundry, pick up a few groceries, or have one of your older children over for a play date.

3. **Consider hiring help.** A postpartum doula (the word is Greek for "woman's servant") is a woman who is specially trained in postpartum care of mothers and newborns. (There are also "birth" doulas who are trained to assist during labor and delivery.) Many doulas have training in breast-

feeding education and some will cook and do light house-keeping, run errands, or care for older children. Doulas are not clinicians; they cannot prescribe medicine, or diagnose medical conditions, but they can be lifesavers during the early postpartum days; they care for you so you can care for your newborn. A doula's fee typically ranges from $15 to $25 per hour, though some charge either a day rate or a flat fee that includes several visits. Some insurance companies will pay for a doula's services.

Questions to Ask a Doula

Before you hire someone to tend to you during this sensitive time, you will want to know a little bit about her. You will want to get recommendations for doulas, as well as conduct the interviews well before your due date. Here are a few questions that you might start with:

- Do you have certification? Who can I call for references?
- Have you had a recent TB test?
- What is your philosophy about parenting and supporting women and their families during the postpartum period?
- What types of services do you provide during the postpartum period?
- If you're not available on a certain day, do you have a partner who will come in your place?
- What are your fees and what do your fees include?

4. **Let Dad handle some of the duties.** Most new dads want to be involved with their new baby's care. You might make him the sole diaperer for the first few days. If your incision is still painful, you will appreciate not having to get up constantly to fetch your baby for feedings if dad is the designated baby delivery guy. With any luck, your partner doted

on you during your pregnancy. We say, let the doting continue. And don't forget to let him know how much you appreciate his efforts.

5. **Practice relaxing.** Alice Domar, PhD, director of the Mind/Body Center at Boston IVF, offers this basic twenty-minute meditation exercise to help bring a sense of physical and mental calm. Sit in a comfortable place. Close your eyes (you can leave them open if you prefer). As you breathe in, silently say a focus word of your choosing (e.g., "One," "Peace," "Shalom," "Heal," "Love"). Draw the sound out. As you exhale, silently say the focus word, or another word that has meaning for you. Inhale through your nose and exhale through your mouth, repeating your words. As you inhale, pause for a few seconds. As you exhale, pause for a few seconds. Repeat a series of in and out breaths ten times. If your mind begins to wander, gently bring it back to your words and focus on your breathing. Don't judge yourself while you meditate; if words or thoughts intrude, gently push them away and focus on your words. When you feel ready, slowly open your eyes, look down for a few moments, and then get up slowly.

Leave well-wishers a message

"After the birth of my son we were overwhelmed by the number of well-wishers who called to check on both of us. Since the baby spent the first few weeks of his life in the hospital, our friends and family would call daily to get the status report—sometimes we got ten or fifteen calls in a day! (We were living far away from home so no one could visit.) For the first couple of days I tried to return all the calls, but it was too much. I realized that no one really wanted to chat, they wanted to know how Liam was doing. One morning I left a message on our machine with an update about Liam's health and that night there was just one message on the machine—from my mom.

Everyone else had listened to the message and then hung up. From that day on, every day before I left for the hospital, I changed the message and left details about our baby's improving health. Even after he came home, we did this for a few weeks until our lives settled down a bit. A postpartum nurse told me she recommends this tip to all her new moms. It can be really hard to get away from feeling obligated to be a good "hostess" during these weeks, but deep down we know what our priorities should be: our own healing and our baby's care."

—Dana, three Cesareans, in 1997, 1999, 2004

CHAPTER 7

Dealing with Mixed Emotions

Delivering by c-section is one road many women are surprised to find themselves traveling down. It can be very unsettling when you're diverted off of one path and forced to go down another that's unknown and maybe even unpleasant.

At some point during your pregnancy, you might have learned that the only way to safely deliver your baby would be by c-section. Maybe you're a first-time mom who attended weeks of childbirth classes that focused intently on preparing you and your partner for a vaginal birth. But things turned out very differently after you went into labor and ultimately delivered by Cesarean. Or perhaps you already have a child and were expecting another vaginal delivery.

A wide range of emotions can surround an unexpected c-section delivery. Feelings of happiness and excitement about the birth of a new baby are undoubtedly high on the list. But you also might have felt anxious, fearful, or even sad upon learning a c-section was necessary. And until you delivered your child, you may not have ever had a reason to be in a hospital, let alone undergo surgery.

While every birth experience is unique, there are many similarities that women who deliver by an unplanned c-section can relate to. Those who found the experience a bit overwhelming probably recall a scenario like this one:

There you were being wheeled into a stark, bright, fluorescent-lit room and placed on an operating table. If you hadn't already been given an epidural, you were asked to roll on to your side or sit up to be given an anesthetic-filled needle in your spine to numb you from the waist down. Or maybe you were given general anesthesia, in which case you don't remember much more after this point. If you are still alert, you begin to feel helpless as your arms are strapped down and an oxygen mask is placed over your mouth and nose to help you breathe. Next, a curtain is draped across your mid-section (if you desired, a mirror was set up so you could watch the surgery). An intravenous needle is inserted into your arm or hand. Little round sticky tabs are pressed on your chest to monitor your vital signs. After the doctor announces she is ready to begin, you feel the sensation of pressure as she makes the first incision. Once the initial cut was made, your obstetrician quickly cuts through several layers of tissue, moving aside your abdominal muscles and bladder in order to get a clear view of your uterus. The uterus is then cut and the amniotic sac ruptured. Soon you feel a very odd, tugging sensation, followed by lots of pressure. Seconds later, your baby is removed from your uterus. But before you can get near your newborn, the pediatrician or attending nurse needs to suction amniotic fluid from his nose and mouth and check his vital signs.

At long last, the nurse brings your baby to you, holding him near your face. Due to the sedative given to help calm you before and during the procedure, you're not allowed to hold the baby unassisted until the medication wears off (most hospitals have this policy). As you see your child for the first time, you smile contently as you stroke his face with your freed hand. But due to the stress of the surgery and the calming drugs that still affect your body, your first

encounter with your newborn isn't quite what you'd antic-
ipated. (We both remembered it as feeling the way you do
when you're halfway through that second glass of wine:
happy, content, but a bit dulled emotionally.) At this point,
your partner and newborn might have left together for the
nursery. Meanwhile, as your OB delivered the placenta,
and began to finish up, you found yourself lying there
thinking: "I went into the delivery room expecting to give
birth to a baby without any major medical intervention,
and now I'm lying on an operating table being sewn back
together!" Snatched from you are those heartwarming
Hollywood images associated with vaginal childbirth: ones
of a sweaty, red-faced, valiant, elated, and overjoyed
woman crossing the finish line and being handed the gold.
(Of course we know very well that in the real world, not all
vaginal births end on this up-note!) Having a c-section,
even if you've labored and pushed for hours, can leave you
feeling as though you've been denied the personal pleasure
of running that last winning mile.

Following the surgery, you were taken to the recovery
room for the next hour or so. If you hadn't done so already,
your whole body might have begun to shake uncontrol-
lably, a reaction to the anesthesia. Slowly, you start to come
out of your surgery-induced fog and regain feeling in your
legs. And right about the time you begin to think you
shouldn't be feeling so sorry for yourself—that you have a
brand-new baby, after all—you proceed to vomit all over
the bedsheets.

Feeling Cheated

It's no wonder that in the minutes, hours, days, and weeks
that follow a c-section, women experience a wide range of emotions. For many, the experience involves hours of labor, surgery,

and the birth of a baby—*all at the same time!* And if you're someone who spent nine months expecting, desiring, and preparing for a vaginal birth, having a c-section can throw you for a loop. It's not unusual to feel as you've somehow failed, or that your doctor, midwife, or labor nurse failed you. Even women who are scheduled for a Cesarean delivery may have been unprepared or distressed by some part of the experience. In addition to failure, you might also be overwhelmed and disappointed, and feel guilt, sadness, fury, rage, and betrayal. "I felt traumatized," is how one woman put it.

Of course, it's important to stress that not all women who deliver by c-section experience negative feelings. In cases where it seems clear that either the mother or baby was at grave risk or the only way to deliver the baby was by Cesarean, a woman may feel relief and gratitude.

Other women we talked with said they didn't have very specific expectations about childbirth. As a result, feelings of inadequacy or disappointment weren't an issue when they wound up having a c-section. For them, having a c-section is seen as another birth option. Lastly, there are growing number of women who welcome the idea of a c-section, preferring to forgo the inconvenience and pains of labor.

Feeling grateful

"I felt blessed to be able to have a c-section. I don't think my daughter would have survived if it wasn't for the surgery. She was up so high and stuck on my pelvic bone, and wasn't going anywhere and my fluid levels were very low. I wonder what would have happened if I didn't have the option of a c-section, like the old days? Would she be alive? Would I? The c-section is what allowed us to safely bring our daughter into the world."

—Christine, mother of one, c-section in 2003

If you had a lot invested in the childbirth experience, from an emotional standpoint, you will find the information that follows both helpful and comforting.

As you spend the next days and weeks physically recovering from the surgery, you may have found your head beginning to swirl with different thoughts and emotions. After a short period, you might have been able to put aside these feelings and not look back. More power to you! But if you're like us and plenty of other women, you could still be grappling with emotional issues surrounding the birth—weeks, months, even years, later. As you rehash the experience in your head, you may wonder: Could something have been done to prevent the surgery? Was it my fault . . . my doctor's . . . the labor nurse's? Will I ever feel normal again? Maybe if I had pushed harder, waited longer before agreeing to a c-section . . . hadn't gained so much weight? When you relay the story of your birth experience to family and friends, you may find yourself trying to justify the need for the surgery, making sure they know just how badly you wanted a vaginal birth, or how many hours of labor you endured or how long you pushed for before you agreed to a c-section.

Not What You Expected

Despite the fact that more than one out of four women in the United States deliver by c-section, many are surprised (especially first-timers) to find themselves undergoing the procedure. Very often, women who attend childbirth classes anticipate having a vaginal birth. Experts say that women who have high expectations about their birth experience may be more prone to negative feelings when things don't turn out the way they'd planned. These are women who like to set goals for themselves and expect to achieve them. When your goal is a vaginal birth, delivering by c-section can feel like a failure.

Of course, you don't have to be goal-oriented to want to experience childbirth that doesn't require cutting your abdomen and uterus open! No one can deny that a desire for a vaginal birth is also largely innate. It's how women have delivered babies for hundreds of thousands of years. We won't argue that, barring any complications involving the mother (including a previous c-section) or child, a vaginal birth is a safer method of delivery for both mother and child, and therefore preferable to a c-section. But the reality is that complications do arise and c-sections become necessary. For this reason, childbirth instructors need to do a better job at educating women about what c-sections entail. Not informing women about their odds of having a c-section birth and what to expect from it because a) they don't support it, and/or b) they think women don't want to hear it, is really ignoring the reality of the statistics. Don't get us wrong, we're not saying that women shouldn't inform their midwives or doctors about their preferences for the things they do have control over. Both of us went into the delivery room with the goal of having a vaginal birth. When we wound up delivering by c-section instead, we felt, like so many of the women we interviewed for this book, caught off guard. After all, we'd left our childbirth classes believing very firmly that how our birth experience went was ultimately within our control. We were sorely misguided. When it comes right down to it, none of us has any real control over whether our babies decide to enter this world head first or feet first, or wind up stuck in the birth canal. So having women believe that they've stayed in control of the birth by not having a c-section, is downright unfair, misleading, and even absurd.

No matter how your opinion about childbirth was shaped, for some, a c-section can be a constant reminder that after nine months of expecting one scenario, things didn't go as you'd planned. Trying to make sense of feelings of disappointment or failure while you also deal with your physical recovery, sleep deprivation, and the demands of caring for a newborn, is enough to make anyone feel overwhelmed! Mental health experts are quick to warn that holding onto or not addressing these negative emotions can damage your emotional, mental, and physical wellbeing. The key to healing, they say, is finding a way to process all of these emotions so that they don't stay bottled up inside.

The Road to Healing

It can take time to process a c-section delivery and accept it for what it is—another birth option. This doesn't mean that you won't always have mixed emotions about the experience, but rather that you've moved beyond the hurt, anger, sadness, or guilt. Getting to this point may take much longer than you want or expect. You can't put a time limit on it. For some, healing comes in a matter of months; for others, years; and still others, never. (We talked with several women who said they were still bothered by their Cesarean deliveries more than a decade later.) Several of the therapists we interviewed for this chapter said that much of a woman's success in dealing with the negative emotions will ultimately come down to how she deals with—or learns to deal with—disappointment, unfairness, and just plain randomness. As one psychologist bluntly put it, "Life sucks sometimes. But part of being a grown-up means you pick yourself up and try to find ways to cope."

So where do you begin? To help answer that, we interviewed four mental health experts who counsel women (and men) on postpartum issues: Deborah Issokson, PsyD, a licensed psychologist and director of Counseling for Reproductive Health & Healing in Watertown, Mass.; Diana Lynn Barnes, PsyD, president of Postpartum Support International, headquartered in Santa Barbara, Calif.; Diane Sanford, PhD, director of the

Women's Healthcare Partnership in St. Louis, Mo.; Shellie Fidell, SCW, a licensed clinical social worker and counselor at the Women's Healthcare Partnership in St. Louis. Here's their advice on helping you come to terms with a Cesarean delivery:

- **Give yourself permission to feel** ... angry, disappointed, pissed-off, confused. You're entitled. Being honest about how the experience has affected you frees you up to begin healing. Suppress or deny the feelings, and therapists say that they'll "leak out" in other ways, like anxiety, depression, overeating, or diminished sex drive.

- **Seek support from family and friends who've had c-sections.** Acknowledging and sharing your feelings with people who love and support you can help you better deal with all the emotions you're experiencing. But follow your gut feelings about whether they share a similar sensibility and philosophy. If you're feeling sad, the last thing you'll want to hear is that your sister-in-law has no regrets about her c-section experience.

- **Join or start a local support group.** Meeting with other women on a regular basis to share your similar experiences is another excellent way to process emotions. Postpartum Support International (PSI) (www.postpartum.net) is an organization that promotes awareness of maternal health issues related to childbearing. They offer resources, referrals, support, and treatment to women and their families who are dealing with postpartum mood disorders. PSI will put you in touch with local support groups or even help you start one in your area.

- **Seek support online.** There are dozens of online support networks and Web sites out there. Many of the pregnant and new mom sites offer c-section message boards or sponsor live chats on the topic. The benefits of using the Internet for support are you don't have to leave your home, you can log on at a time convenient for you, and you can remain anonymous, if that makes you more comfortable. The downside, warn therapists, is that getting hooked on them can sometimes perpetuate the problem.

- **Find a framework for healing that suits you.** You might do better with a spiritual angle, like meditating, or opt for the intellectual and choose to read up on everything related to c-sections and why they happen. One or more approaches could work for you. The key is finding out which best suits your personality.

- **Know that it's okay to feel conflicting emotions.** After a c-section, it's quite normal to feel polar emotions. For instance, you might be thrilled about your newborn baby and at the same time extremely disappointed about not having a vaginal birth. But even though it's common to experience such a wide range of feelings, don't expect to get a lot of support. Mental health experts say that our culture tends to reject the idea of conflicting feelings—you're happy or sad, not both. People, in general, can also be uncomfortable hearing that you're sad, depressed, or angry. Many women feel compelled to put on a happy face and claim everything is just fine, when things are far from okay. Ultimately, suppressing such negative emotions can lead to anxiety, depression, or destructive behavior, such as alcohol or drug abuse.

. . . .

Conflicting emotions

"I definitely felt disappointed following my c-section birth, but I rarely felt free to admit that because so often people will say, 'Well, what really matters is that you had a healthy baby.' Duh. It's very hard to find someone who can understand that it's possible to separate those two issues in your mind, to know that having the c-section is the safest thing to do, but to still be disappointed in missing out on the birth experience."

—Maura, mother of three, one c-section in 1990

- **Express yourself in writing.** If you're comfortable writing, use a journal to express your thoughts, gripes, etc. Consider writing a letter to yourself or your child about the birth experience. You could talk about how things went or even how you'd wish they'd gone. If you're unhappy with the way your midwife, obstetrician, or nurse handled the birth, you might send each of them a letter citing your grievances. (But realize that if you should decide to actually mail the letters, it doesn't mean you'll get a positive—or any—response.) The act of writing will help you to sort through problematic issues and release negative feelings.

  As for how often and how much you should write, it's up to you. Some people like to journal just a few times a week, for an hour or more, while others write daily for just a few minutes. But since a lot of what you're writing about may be negative, consider starting a separate "gratefulness" journal to help shift your energy to a more positive realm. Write about things that inspire you, make you laugh, feel good, happy, lucky, loved, and thankful you're alive. Then make a point to read the journal at least once a week.

- **Exercise your inner Picasso.** If writing doesn't suit you, try expressing yourself by painting, sculpting, drawing, even doing crafts—you get the picture. Using art as a form of release can be very powerful in your healing.

- **Reframe the experience.** Putting a frame around what did go well with the birth can be very empowering. Maybe the operation was complication-free and you felt a lot less pain than you'd expected. Or maybe the hospital staff went out of their way to make you comfortable during your stay. Perhaps your family and friends rallied to support you during your recovery.

- **Tell yourself that there is no right or wrong way to deliver a baby.** Looking at your c-section delivery as though it's simply an alternative birthing method, and not secondary to a vaginal birth, can help you feel more accepting of your delivery experience. This acceptance will allow you to reach the point where you can let go of all the negative feelings associated with your c-section.

- **Work on healing your body, too.** Just as important as healing your mind is restoring your body. Not surprisingly, many women feel out of sync with their bodies after undergoing abdominal surgery. You can also feel let down by your body since it wasn't able to birth a baby vaginally. Taking steps to restore your body—whether that means rebuilding your abs or doing exercises like kickboxing, Pilates, swimming, or yoga—can really facilitate total body healing. (For more, see Chapter Nine, "Body Wellness.") One woman we talked with said it was the challenge of training for and running a marathon that allowed her to reclaim her body following her Cesarean.

- **Realize when it's time to move on.** In order to achieve healing, there is a point at which you finally have to let go. You have to make a choice about how you want to progress from a traumatic event. How you get meaning from your experience might mean drawing on things like friends or religion.

Moving on doesn't have to mean that you've completely accepted what has happened. While some women might eventually feel that they've reached a point of total healing, for others, their c-section experience will always remain a sore spot. In either case, moving ahead means that you've gotten to a place where the experience no longer takes center stage in your daily thinking. What propels you to that place really depends on how you choose to cope. Some may benefit simply from following the preceding advice, while others will need the additional support of professional counseling. As for *when* the healing happens, sometimes a new life event (the birth of another child, a new job) helps you to move on; in other cases, the healing takes place over time as you develop a relationship with your child and grow as a family. During this journey of recovery, it's important to remember that there is no single way to heal and no specific timetable for healing.

- **Seek professional help if you don't feel better.** If you find yourself consumed with negative feelings about your c-section, or you're not sleeping or eating, or you're feeling really down and experience a deep sense of hopelessness, it's time to talk to a professional who can help you sort through things and get you the help you need. Many medical insurance companies provide mental health services for their members and can help you find a therapist.

Sound Familiar?

While researching the book we discovered that many women shared some of same self-defeating feelings—either initially or long-term—about their c-section birth experiences. We've included several of these sentiments below, along with advice on how to counter the negative statements:

"I feel like less of a mother because I didn't birth my baby vaginally."

The reality: There are many different ways that we become mothers—through a marriage, adoption, a vaginal birth. And while a vaginal birth may be the desirable method of delivering a baby for a lot of women, having a baby by Cesarean section certainly doesn't mean you're any less of a mother. The real test of how much of a mother you are begins with how you choose to raise your child. Remember, labor and childbirth can last for a day or two. You will be a mother forever.

"I feel like my body let me down."

The reality: You could be the strongest, most fit woman on the planet and *still* have a Cesarean birth. Childbirth is a complicated miracle with so many variables, most of which are out of your control. Delivering a baby vaginally has nothing to do with how far you can run, how many sit-ups you can do, or how many colds you *don't* catch in a given year. Look at it this way: your body actually grew that baby, and up to the moment of his first breath, your body kept your child alive.

"This baby doesn't really feel like he's mine since I didn't feel a thing, or I wasn't even coherent."

The reality: Not being an active physical participant in the birth process does make you feel somewhat removed from the whole experience. But there are ways to try to reconnect. If you did feel movement and pressure as the baby was being removed from your uterus, try to focus on those feelings. If you were completely knocked out, viewing pictures or videotape, or having your doctor or partner recount the birth, can help.

"I feel horrible because I wasn't overjoyed upon seeing my baby for the first time."

The reality: The stress and fatigue that results from the surgery along with the emotion-numbing painkillers can leave you physically and emotionally drained. If you had an emergency c-section, just trying to process that independently of everything else can be overwhelming. Chances are that once the drugs wore off and you got some rest you were smiling from ear to ear upon seeing your baby. And remember: women who birth their babies vaginally aren't always overcome with joy upon seeing their baby for the first time either. After hours of labor and pushing, some are too tired to even want to hold the baby.

The first meeting

"Before I gave birth I thought I'd be bawling and so happy when I first saw my child. But the whole thing seemed very surreal. My arms were strapped down, so I didn't get to hold him right away. And I remember thinking, why didn't I cry when I first saw him? I felt guilty afterward for not being happy."

—Carole, mother of one, c-section in 2001

"We didn't get to bond properly because we were separated for hours after the birth."

The reality: Childbirth instructors and pregnancy books do a real disservice by overstressing the importance of the first few minutes and hours after birth. You will be bonding with your child every day until he leaves for college! Trust us, you won't love your baby any less and he won't love you any less because you didn't get to hold him until he was a few hours old. And if for some reason he ended up in the neonatal intensive care unit (as one of our babies did), you will have plenty of opportunities to make up for lost time in the months and years to come.

"After all the trouble I had with infertility, I should just be happy that I have a baby."

The reality: Again, there's another myth that just because you struggled with infertility you shouldn't have any emotional attachments to how your baby is born. Like any woman, you're perfectly entitled to desire a vaginal birth. Likewise, you're perfectly entitled to feel disappointment when that doesn't happen. But ultimately, it's important that you accept your birth experience for what it was.

"If only I had . . .

. . . **pushed harder.**" The reality: You could have pushed for three days and the baby might never have come out. Some babies' heads are simply too big to fit into the birth canal.

. . . **waited longer.**" The reality: Many doctors operate on the premise that when it comes to childbirth, things can go from good to bad very quickly. Cognitive rationalization on their part is integral to deciding whether there is imminent risk for you or your baby. Add the threat of a malpractice suit and you can see why, when labor isn't progressing as it should, some docs opt for a Cesarean sooner rather than later. Hopefully, you feel you can trust your doctor's decision making. If not, there may be issues to resolve with your doctor.

. . . **not gained so much weight.**" The reality: It's true that gaining more than the recommended twenty-five to thirty-five pounds increases your chances of delivering by c-section. There are a few reasons this is so: the more weight you gain, the bigger the baby. The bigger the baby, the harder it is for the baby to get through the canal. Maternal obesity also has associated health risks, including high blood pressure, heart disease, and diabetes, conditions for which Cesarean delivery is often indicated. But eating nutritiously and getting exercise doesn't guarantee that you won't have a c-section.

. . . **not had an epidural.**" The reality: The jury is still out on this one. While there seems to be a relationship between epidurals and c-sections, there's no proof that one causes the other. More accurately, women who request epidurals may be experiencing more difficult labors, and a difficult labor is more likely to end with a c-section delivery.

"I feel like a failure."

Not every woman who's had a c-section will feel like a failure. In fact, as we've said before, some women aren't emotionally invested in how their baby will be born. And there are even some women who prefer a c-section to a vaginal birth. But for women who have c-sections and feel as though somehow they've failed, experts say that it's okay to mourn not having a vaginal birth. But ranking one method of delivery as better or more worthy than the other only sets you up for negative feelings.

. . . .

Justifying a Cesarean

"My Bradley Method childbirth instructor called a few weeks after the birth to see how we'd done. I told her what happened: I had pushed for two excruciating hours before it was clear that Jack wasn't going to come out any other way but through my belly. When I was finished sharing the story of my c-section she said . . . nothing.

"Her silence made me feel like I'd failed myself and my child. In the weeks following my son's birth, I was overwhelmed, in pain, and having trouble getting my baby to nurse. As the months passed, my feelings only intensified. When I went to playgroups, I'd listen to my friends sharing their vaginal birth stories while I just sat and thought, 'Wow, I really screwed up.' I felt like I had to offer up a minute-by-minute description of my labor in order to 'justify' my Cesarean."

—Maureen, mother of two, c-sections in 1999 and 2001

. . . .

"I could never, ever do this again."

One of us couldn't imagine undergoing another c-section after her first experience—the post-op gas pains alone were enough to stop at one child. But like millions of women, we both got pregnant again, and had c-sections again. Therapists says that it's important to censor your self-narratives. In this case, try distinguishing what's true about the statement and what's not true. "I could *never* do this again" is quite different from "I really don't want to do this again."

Postpartum Depression and/or Anxiety

Can having a c-section make you more prone to postpartum depression? Research from one study conducted at Alliant International University-California School of Professional Psychology in San Diego involving 107 women showed that those who had unexpected c-sections were most likely to experience symptoms of depression when compared with women who had planned c-sections or vaginal deliveries. Interestingly, among the three groups, the planned c-sections reported the fewest symptoms of depression.

Researchers say that it's not entirely clear whether an unplanned c-section in and of itself can lead to depression, or if it's that women who are prone to depression are more likely to suffer from it following one. Genetics, biology, and hormones all play a role in who is affected by depression. In many instances, your emotional response to an unexpected situation and how you choose to deal with it depend on how you handle disappointment, how traumatic the experience was, and how much support you get once you're home.

No matter what your birth experience is, 50–80 percent of new mothers develop some form of the "baby blues." Because it occurs with such frequency, it is not considered a mental health disorder. Symptoms, which usually crop up around day three and dissipate by day fourteen, include tearfulness, anxiety, exhaustion, and mood instability. Rapid hormonal changes along with the physical and emotional stress of birthing contribute to the blues. Generally, most women are able to manage their symptoms with adequate rest, good nutrition, and lots of support and reassurance from family and friends. Psychological treatment is not usually necessary for these women.

Knowing the signs of postpartum depression and when to seek help for it is critical to your and your baby's well-being.

As many as 20 percent of women experience postpartum depression with symptoms ranging from mild to severe. After two weeks, the feelings mentioned earlier will persist and start to intensify. Despite being exhausted, you may not be able to sleep. You may experience changes in appetite. You may feel confused and unable to concentrate—"in a fog" is how many women describe it. We're not talking about the fogginess you feel from lack of sleep or from the painkillers. When it's depression, the fog dulls everything around you.

Other symptoms can include memory loss, and feeling scared, terribly anxious, and overwhelmed by the responsibilities of taking care of your infant. You might also feel emotionally detached from your infant, irritable, and short-tempered. Feelings of inadequacy often surface as some women begin to question their maternal competency and actually see themselves as replaceable. Women with severe depression may consider suicide. On top of it, you may feel ashamed of how you're feeling and be afraid of being alone with the baby.

Getting Help

Very often, women are willing to tolerate an awful lot, suffering in silence before they ask for help. In moderate to severe cases of depression, or with psychosis (mentioned later), medical intervention is essential to recovery. Treatment usually involves a combination of counseling, aka "talk therapy," and the use of antidepressant medications. Drugs such as Prozac, Zoloft, Effexor, and Celexa are often used in combination with antianxiety medications like Ativan and Xanax. The course of treatment is usually twelve to eighteen months, depending on depression history and severity, and duration of symptoms. For those who are breast-feeding, Zoloft and Paxil are the top choices because studies show that little or none of the medication is detected in breast milk.

Postpartum Psychosis

Postpartum psychosis is rare, affecting one of every 1,000 women who give birth. Symptoms come on suddenly at day three or four and can include hearing voices, obsessive thoughts, and delusional thinking (for example, feeling directed to kill your baby). A woman with this illness tends to isolate herself and withdraw. This condition is a life-threatening medical emergency that requires immediate hospitalization. Since a woman experiencing this disorder will not recognize it, her partner, spouse, or other family member must assist her in getting the help she desperately needs.

Post-Traumatic Stress Disorder

In some cases, an emergency Cesarean can trigger Post-Traumatic Stress Disorder (PTSD). The psychological stress of the surgery can set off a host of symptoms: flashbacks to the birth experience, tremendous anxiety, recurrent nightmares, hypervigilance in caring for your baby, feelings of doom. Those who are prone to anxiety disorders may be more prone to PTSD. Sometimes, but not always, there is an unresolved early childhood trauma, such as physical or sexual abuse, which can also make you more likely to develop the condition. You don't have to suffer with these symptoms. Finding a therapist who treats this disorder is the first step toward healing. (The American Association of Marriage and Family Therapy [www.aamft.org] and the American Psychological Association [www.apa.org] have Web sites that can help you with your search.) Treatment involves a combination of psychotherapy and antidepressant medication.

CHAPTER 8

Concerns and Questions Your Partner Might Have

Y ou have just learned that your wife or partner will deliver your baby by Cesarean. Or maybe she's still in the hospital following a Cesarean birth. Now you're wondering what it means for her, and what it means for the baby.

For starters, you probably have many questions about the procedure: What are the risks? What will the recovery involve? Here we'll answer the most common ones.

Frequently Asked Questions . . .

. . . Before a C-Section

Q. **Can I be with my wife or partner in the operating room?**

A. If this is a scheduled surgery or an unplanned, nonemergency procedure, you can accompany your partner in the operating room for the entire time. You'll be asked to put on scrubs (a surgical top and pants, a cap, and sterile mask). You'll sit near your partner's head and be able to touch her face or hands.

In the case of a true emergency—meaning your partner's or baby's life is at risk—you'll need to wait outside the operating room. The reason: the surgical team wants to be sure any complications are under control first. They also want to protect you from witnessing what could be a traumatic event. Once it's clear that things are okay they may allow you to come in just before the baby is about to be born. In some cases, the surgical attendants may be too busy or distracted to walk out and invite you back in. If it's been more than twenty minutes and you haven't heard from anyone, ask to talk to the "charge" nurse on that floor. She's the person in charge of that particular shift in that unit. She should be able to find out whether you can enter the operating room and help you scrub and get changed into sterile clothing so that you can go into the OR.

Q. **How long will the procedure take?**

A. The average c-section takes around forty-five minutes from the time of the initial incision. But there are certain circumstances that can extend the procedure. If your partner has had a previous Cesarean, or other abdominal surgery, it may take the physician a few extra minutes to make the initial incisions since she has to cut through existing scar tissue. If your partner develops a complication such as excessive bleeding, it may add some time to the surgery while the physician and her assistants work to get the bleeding under control. And if your partner is delivering more than one baby, that will also add some time to the procedure.

Q. **Will my wife or partner feel much pain during the procedure?**

A. No, she shouldn't feel any pain. In approximately 90 percent of cases, a woman is given regional anesthesia by injection in the lower spine. This type of anesthesia numbs her from the lower chest down, but allows her to be awake and alert throughout the surgery. She may experience a tugging sensation—most likely when the baby is being pulled from her uterus.

In 8 to 11 percent of Cesarean deliveries, general anesthesia is required. This type of pain medication is administered through a combination of inhaled gases and intra-venous drugs. Since she is not awake during the procedure, she is unable to feel pain.

Q. **Is there any risk to her? The baby?**

A. Like any surgery, there are always risks. Fortunately, serious complications involving c-sections are rare. Problems that can arise during the actual surgery include hemorrhaging (uncontrollable bleeding) and injury to the bowels or blad-der. Following a c-section there is a risk of postpartum in-fection and blood clots, but these complications are rare.

The risks to the baby are also minimal. Even with all the technology we have—from sonograms that measure the baby's height and weight to amniocentesis that can be used to check lung development—babies still occasionally get delivered by Cesarean too soon. When that happens, the baby can face a host of problems associated with incomplete lung development and prematurity. Babies born by Cesarean are also at a higher risk of developing some respiratory problems, and physicians think that because they don't experience the natural onset of labor, they miss out on some of the hormones that help them prepare their lungs for breathing outside of the womb. Generally these problems are minor and require minimal treatment, such as extra suctioning and supplemental oxygen.

Q. **Can I videotape or take pictures during the surgery?**

A. It depends on the policies of your hospital. Most hospitals allow you to videotape and take pictures once the baby is born, including that thrilling moment when the physician presents your baby to the world. But filming and photo-graphing the actual surgery are usually prohibited. When your baby is ready to be born the obstetrician will alert you so you can get ready with your equipment.

Q. Can I still cut the umbilical cord?

A. Usually, no. But if this is very important to you, you may ask if there is any way an exception can be made. Because you and your wife are not "sterile"—meaning you haven't scrubbed up for the surgery—and you will probably be sitting with her, it would be too risky for you to then move into a sterile field where you would expose mom to potentially harmful bacteria.

Q. Will I be able to hold the baby as soon as he's born?

A. In most cases, yes. However, even if all signs indicate your baby is okay, you may still have to wait five minutes or so before your baby is handed to you. In many situations the pediatrician will need to suction any amniotic fluid from his nose and mouth, assess his breathing and overall health, and then wrap the baby in blankets or place him in a warming bassinet or under heat lamps.

After you and your partner have had a chance to hold your newborn, a nurse will place him in a transporter (a bassinet with wheels) to bring him to the nursery. If you choose to go with your baby to the nursery, you'll get to observe the nurse while she weighs and measures him and gives him his first bath. But realize that once you leave the OR to go to the nursery, you won't be permitted back in. The operating room is a sterile area and the nursery is not. You'll need to wait until your partner is in the recovery area before seeing her again. If for some reason your baby was in distress or showed other signs of impairment, he'll be attended to in the operating room and then taken to the neonatal intensive care unit where the nurses and pediatrician or neonatalogist can monitor him. Unless your baby's health is in jeopardy, you will be able to accompany him to the nursery.

. . . *After the Procedure*

Q. How much pain will she be in afterward?

A. Many physicians have begun administering a onetime, intravenous dose of morphine toward the end of the surgery. This does a great job of controlling pain for the next eighteen to twenty-four-hours. Once the morphine wears off, your partner will be given either injectable pain medication, oral painkillers, or an intravenous pump that allows her to self-administer her medication. These medicines also do a good job of controlling pain. After a few days she'll be able to take a less potent pain medication such as nonprescription strength ibuprofen (Advil). Even when she's on pain medication, for the first two days or so she will be very sore and may have difficulty getting out of bed and moving around.

Q. How long will she stay in the hospital?

A. The average stay following a c-section surgery is four days, including the day of the delivery. By law your partner is entitled to ninety-six hours of in-hospital care following a c-section. Certain things, such as postpartum infection, may make it necessary to prolong the stay. On the other hand, some women choose to leave earlier than the expected four days. (If your partner elects to leave early, remember that for the next several days she will need extra help. Even the most mundane tasks, like taking a shower, can be challenging following surgery. It's up to you to make sure that she doesn't overdo it.)

Q. Will I be allowed to visit my partner and baby whenever I want?

A. Many hospitals allow partners to stay in the room and also encourage that the baby room-in with mom. If your partner is sharing a room with another patient, to respect her privacy, the hospital may ask that you leave at 11 p.m. and not arrive before 9 a.m.

Q. How long will her recovery be?

A. The recovery period is about six weeks. During this time your partner will be restricted from vigorous physical activity. This means no exercise other than walking and some gentle stretches, no heavy lifting—nothing heavier than your baby—since it puts pressure on her incision and interferes with healing. For the first ten days to two weeks she'll be discouraged from driving. If she's taking any pain medication, her reaction time will be slowed, making it dangerous for her to be on the road. Her incision may make it difficult to step on the brakes with force. Plus, if she's driving, it's likely that she's not resting as much as she should be. During her first two weeks home, she should try to limit the number of times she climbs stairs because this puts additional strain on her incision. Same goes for regular household chores, like laundry and vacuuming.

Q. Will she still be able to take care of the baby?

A. Yes, although initially she may need help with picking up the baby, diaper changes, and bottle preparation. One way you can help limit extra trips up and down stairs, or just up and down the hall, is to set up a temporary diaper-changing station near your partner's side of the bed. You can either move the changing table into your bedroom for the first few weeks, or just gather all the diaper-changing supplies and put them in a basket next to your bed. Don't forget to include a stack of towels to serve as changing pads, and a diaper pail, which you can be in charge of emptying every day.

Q. She really wants to breast-feed. Will she still be able to?

A. Yes. The surgery may make it more of a challenge due to the gas pains and soreness from the incision, but these will soon dissipate and she will be able to nurse comfortably. The painkillers that she'll be given at the hospital will also help her to nurse without a lot of pain. These are considered safe to take while breast-feeding. There are only a few medications that are not recommended for nursing moms and they include lithium (for manic depressive illness), methotrexate (for arthritis), bromocriptine (for Parkinson's disease), most chemotherapy drugs, and ergotamine (for migraines).

Q. How can I help?

A. The best thing you can do is encourage your partner to rest as much as possible the first two weeks that she's home. You can arrange for outside help from friends and family (especially if you need to be back at work and/or have older children to care for) during this two-week period. After that, she can start to resume some normal activities like doing household chores, cooking, and driving, and participating in the day-to-day care of the baby and other children. But she still won't be 100 percent, so if at all possible, arrange to be home early some days or even take a day off here and there.

Q. Will her scar be noticeable?

A. If she had the abdominal incision known as the bikini cut, it'll be barely noticeable once it's healed. This scar sits just above the pubic bone and is about four inches long. Most women are bothered more by the little pouch of tummy fat that now hangs above the scar. If your partner had a vertical incision, the scar will be much more visible because it'll run up the center of her abdomen.

Q. Other than the scar, are there lasting effects from the surgery?

A. In some cases, internal scar tissue can adhere to the abdominal wall or other organs and cause problems such as intermittent pain or interfere with egg implantation in future attempts to get pregnant. With future pregnancies, there is always the risk of uterine rupture due to her weakened uterus. But, again, this is an infrequent occurrence and something her physician will keep a close eye on. Some women do have lasting emotional effects from a c-section surgery—especially when they weren't expecting it or very much desired a vaginal birth.

Q. How soon until we can have sex?

A. Her doctor will recommend that she not have intercourse until she's gone two weeks without bleeding, which will probably be around six weeks following the surgery.

Don't forget she's had a c-section

"I had a tendency to forget that my wife just had major surgery. Everyone was so happy and joyous about the baby, but here was my wife who, two days later, could still only walk by taking baby steps because she was so uncomfortable from being cut open."

—Tim, father of one son born in 2003

How You Can Help at Home

Once home, you play a critical role in helping your partner to heal. That includes being there for her on an emotional and practical level. Some quick tips:

- **Consider taking some more time off.** If you weren't expecting a c-section delivery, you may have only taken a week or so off from work. Having you home for at least two weeks (if not longer) will be a big help to your partner. Even if you have other relatives staying with you, no one knows your wife better than you do. (Okay, maybe her mother or best friend have a good pulse on it, but they're still not the same as you, the new dad.)

- **Set up a mode for communication.** If you live in a two-floor dwelling and your partner plans on setting up camp in the second floor bedroom for the first few days or so, do yourself a favor and outfit yourselves with some type of communication device. Cell phones, two-way walkie-talkies, or even a baby monitor will come in handy when your spouse needs a refill on her water, gets hungry, or needs help with the baby.

- **Ask her what she needs from you.** Maybe she'd rather her mother run to the grocery store for diapers, and have you sit with her while she nurses and changes the baby or you eat lunch together. If fetching baby from the nursery is wearing her out, be willing to bring the baby to her for feedings after changing his diaper. Taking part in the day-to-day care of your newborn is the best way to forge a bond.

- **Make sure she gets enough fluids and food.** Fluids and nutritious food are essential to any woman's recovery from surgery and childbirth. If your spouse has chosen to breast-feed, these two things are even more critical to maintaining her energy level and breast milk production. Ask her for recommendations on what types of foods she'd like for each of her meals. Consider stocking a cooler full of bottled water and snacks (such as fruit, dry cereal, cheese sticks, and crackers) so she has easy access.

- **Be prepared to pamper.** You know what your partner likes, and there's no better time to indulge her than during the first few weeks postpartum. Does she like aromatherapy? Find some special candles or lotions that she can enjoy during her recovery. Does she like to have her hair brushed? Enjoy back massages? These little acts of love go a long way toward making your partner feel better.

The Ultimate Foot Massage

If your partner considers a foot massage the ultimate act of love, here's one you can try (we learned it at a spa in New York City):

1. Encircle her foot in both hands and, with light pressure, slide your hands on the top-side of her foot, working from the toes up toward the ankle and then back down. Increase the pressure with each upward stroke but lighten your grip on the way down. This will also help reduce swelling that often occurs during pregnancy and afterward. Do this ten times.

2. Cradle the foot near her ankle with one hand. Using the thumb on your other hand, slide it between the bones that run from each toe to the ankle, starting at the toe end. Increase pressure slightly as you move upward. Repeat.

3. Cup the foot in one hand and use the thumb and forefinger of the other hand to gently pinch the Achilles tendon, starting at the heel and moving down toward the ankle. Then, using light pressure, "draw" twenty circles around the ankle bones with your thumbs. Rotate the ankle one way and then the other.

4. Holding the foot in one hand, make a fist with the other and slide the flat surface—between the first two joints of your fingers—firmly along the heel, sole, and ball of the foot. Rotate your fist as you go back and forth several times.

5. Encircle the foot with both hands; press firmly with your thumbs, start at the heel and move up toward the ball of the foot.

6. Take one foot in one hand and gently pull one toe at a time, then roll each one between your fingers.

7. Repeat from step one on the other foot.

Not what I expected

"Up until the surgery, my wife and I had been experiencing the labor together—timing the contractions at home, the drive to the hospital, my holding her hand in the birthing room. I felt like I was really of part of what was happening. But when they decided our first son would have to be born by Cesarean, I had to go put on a surgical cap and gown and then wait for a few minutes before I could go into the operating room. I remember sitting alone and thinking 'My whole life is in that room.' It was a very helpless, scary feeling."

—John, father of two boys born by Cesarean in 1999 and 2001

The Unexpected C-Section

The unexpected c-section can be an overwhelming experience for you, too. If this is your first child, there's a good chance you recently attended a birthing class to prepare you and your partner for a vaginal delivery. But then the birth experience turned out to be completely different. Instead of being in the role of the trusted labor coach, you were relegated to the sidelines and left to stand by and observe (or wait anxiously outside the operating room) while your wife required surgery to deliver your baby.

David Diamond, PhD, director of The Center for Reproductive Psychology, a nonprofit organization affiliated with Alliant International University-California School of Professional Psychology in San Diego, says that many partners are also invested in a particular kind of birth experience, just like the woman giving birth is. On some level you could be trying to come to grips with the loss of a vaginal delivery, too.

Unlike the woman, however, the man is typically less likely to be consciously aware of a "loss." While all men will respond differently depending on their personalities, says Diamond, in general, men often feel as though they should be in control and be able to manage their feelings. It's not unusual for you to become impatient with your wife or partner for being emotional about the Cesarean. Realize that being impatient may be less about intolerance and more about not wanting your wife or partner to remind you of what you're trying *not* to feel.

And just because you're not talking about the experience to friends and family the way your partner is, it doesn't mean that you weren't affected or that you don't care. Throwing yourself into work or projects at home might be your way of dealing with a situation that didn't work out the way you'd hoped.

In cases when the birth is a traumatic experience—the baby or mother's life was at risk, they were harmed, or there is loss of life—you, like your partner, can develop symptoms of depression or post-traumatic stress disorder (PTSD). For men the symptoms of depression can include an inability to concentrate at work or home, exhaustion, a change in appetite, and mood instability. In cases of PTSD, you may have recurrent nightmares about the experience, flashbacks, frightening images, and a sense of doom. In either of these situations, it's important to seek help from a licensed therapist who can help you sort out your issues by talking about the experience, and, if necessary, prescribe medication.

Why Can't She Just Move On?

When your spouse or partner has a hard time accepting a c-section delivery or wants to talk about it frequently, you might find yourself struggling to understand where she's coming from.

Deborah Issokson, PsyD, a licensed psychologist and director of Counseling for Reproductive Health & Healing in Watertown, Mass., says it's important for men to understand that following a birth, women take on a new social identity. As a mother of a new baby, a woman is constantly being asked to relate her birth story to just about everyone she encounters. She's asked to field well-meaning questions, like: How'd things go? Did you have an easy time of it? Was it a vaginal birth? Did you go for the drugs? As a result, your wife or partner is forced to constantly review the events that took place. And when things didn't go as planned, she may also feel the need to defend what happened. On a more positive note, a woman may use talking as a way to process the events.

But what can happen for men, says Issokson, is that at some point you get sick of hearing about it, mostly because the birth experience (not to be confused with your child) just doesn't hold as much meaning to you. Try to be patient throughout this time and to gain a better understanding of where she's coming from by putting yourself in her place.

If after two weeks following the delivery your spouse has become consumed with the topic or starts to show signs of depression (symptoms can include feelings of hopelessness, mood instability, chronic insomnia, a change of eating habits), let her know that she doesn't need to suffer alone with these feelings. A combination of mental health counseling, and possibly medication, can get her back on track. (For more on postpartum depression, see Chapter 7, "Dealing with Mixed Emotions.")

CHAPTER 9

Body Wellness

"My incision is so red and my whole belly is puffy . . . will it always look like this? . . . I'm not pregnant anymore, but from the side I still look it and I still need to wear my maternity jeans! . . . How can I exercise if I'm worried I'll split my incision open every time I move? . . . Sex? Forget it!"

Yep. We know exactly what you're thinking. And the information we've compiled for this chapter and the one that follows, "The Ultimate Post–C-Section Workout," will help you take the first steps back to fitness (and intimacy). But we can't proceed without a gentle reminder that it took nine months to grow your baby and you can't expect every trace of your pregnancy—Cesarean scar included—to disappear within nine days or nine weeks of delivery. In fact, it may take nine months or more until you are able to fit back into your "regular" clothes or return to your prepregnancy fitness level.

If that sounds like an impossibly long time, consider the position that one renowned pregnancy-and-exercise expert takes: "The definition of the postpartum period should be extended to *one year* because many of the physiological changes from pregnancy exist at least that long," says Michelle Mottola, PhD, a Canadian exercise scientist who helped develop the Canadian health system's pregnancy exercise guidelines. Whenever you're feeling frustrated by how you look, try this little trick: pick up your baby and walk to the nearest mirror. Look at yourself while you're holding him in your arms and tell yourself the truth: *you have never looked better!* It's hard to be critical of your body when you're holding a newborn in your arms.

Now we'll get to the point. You already know the reasons that exercise is important, but some of them are worth repeating. Consistent exercise lowers your risk of breast cancer, colon cancer, heart disease, osteoporosis, and diabetes. (One of the greatest gifts you can give your child is your own healthy longevity.) Exercise also reduces body fat, something that is generally at the top of the list for a woman who's just had a baby. That's one reason we were surprised to find that when it comes to postpartum exercise advice, there isn't much out there.

One physician, a woman who had her own babies via Cesarean, told us that most physicians who care for women during pregnancy think their work ends once the pregnancy ends. She put it like this: "The baby has been born, so the doctor says to the new mom, 'I've done *my* job, now *you* figure out the rest.'" When asked about the best kinds of exercise we could do after our Cesareans, one of our physicians said, "Just use common sense." He was well-meaning, of course, but that wasn't the most helpful advice. In all fairness to the OB/GYNs—physicians who generally aren't fitness experts—there isn't much scientific research that has looked at exercise during the postpartum period, so there simply aren't many specific recommendations that they can offer. Yet one group of researchers who investigated issues facing women during the postpartum period found that at seven weeks postpartum, 75 percent of the study's participants wanted more information about one of the topics that their physician discussed with them at their checkup. *The highest percentage of them wanted more information on exercise, diet, and nutrition.*

If you exercised throughout your pregnancy, you are probably anxious to get back into a routine. If you didn't, there is nothing like those leftover pregnancy pounds to motivate you to start now. We know very well that finding the time and energy to exercise once there's a baby in the picture can be a challenge. But the benefits are so great that we can't think of any good reason you shouldn't try to work in at least some form of exercise. We recommend you check with your healthcare provider before you begin any kind of exercise that is more strenuous than walking, or requires that you lift anything heavier than your baby. Because of your Cesarean delivery, you do need to take more precautions—and ease into any exercise program more slowly—than someone who had an uncomplicated vaginal delivery.

First Things First: Get Moving ASAP

As you learned in previous chapters, one of the best things you can do for yourself during the early days of recovery from your Cesarean is to get out of bed and get moving. The nurses who cared for you in the hospital should have encouraged you to get out of bed and walk within twelve to eighteen hours of your surgery, if not sooner. Getting on your feet improves digestion, decreases muscle stiffness, and lowers your risk of developing blood clots; *movement is vital to your healing.* As you did in the hospital, try to support your incision with your hands or a pillow during these first days. You may feel like you don't want to walk, but getting over this hurdle is the first step to getting your body back.

Walking, deep breathing, and gentle stretches and even some basic exercises will not pull apart your incision. This kind of light activity will help you heal because it improves circulation, which in turn promotes healing. Even if all you can do at first is walk for five minutes once around the block, so be it. That's a start!

Fatigue is certainly your constant companion these days, and walking will actually improve your energy level. Women who exercise during the postpartum period have been shown to be more likely to have positive moods, are less anxious and depressed, and have increased energy after exercise. Be aware that although you had a surgical delivery, you will still have some vaginal bleeding because the placenta has detached from the uterus and the "placental site" must heal. There is no evidence, however, that exercise after childbirth increases normal bleeding after delivery or increases the risk of postpartum hemorrhage. Even though the advice to use common sense isn't exactly—well—exact, you should pay close attention to your body as you embark on your exercise program, especially during these early days. If something doesn't feel right, or if bleeding increases significantly, it's better to back off for a few days than to jeopardize your healing.

A Word of Caution

The following exercises are very gentle, but we urge you to talk with your physician before you begin. If you had a complicated delivery, or lost a significant amount of blood, she may discourage you from doing anything other than Kegel exercises and taking very short walks for a few weeks.

Starting Day 1: Continue Your Kegels and Take a Breathing Lesson

During your pregnancy, your healthcare provider and your childbirth educator probably stressed the importance of doing daily perineal or pelvic floor strengthening exercises. The pelvic floor is really a group of three muscles and the connective tissues around the vagina and anus. Among other things, these muscles control the flow of urine. The pelvic floor also supports all of the organs—including the bladder and uterus—that sit between the tailbone and the pubic bone. Even though you didn't have a vaginal birth, pregnancy (not to mention aging) takes a toll on these muscles.

Doing Kegels will help you maintain strength in your pelvic floor, and reduce the chances of experiencing urinary incontinence. Plus, you can do them within hours of your surgery and you can do them anywhere.

The best way to start with Kegels is simply to contract the muscles that surround the opening of the urethra, vagina, and anus and hold the contraction for about ten seconds and repeat ten to twenty times. Aim to do this three times throughout the day. A more advanced type of Kegel is called the "elevator." To do this exercise, tighten the muscles of your sphincter and then try to "lift" up between your rectum and vagina. Lift as high as you can and then hold for three to five seconds and then release very slowly, one "floor" at a time. You'll find that as your pelvic muscles get stronger, you'll have more control and be able to release more slowly. Try this exercise six times a day.

You can also do some deep breathing exercises starting on Day 1. Breathing deeply will help cleanse your lungs of residual anesthesia and reduce risk for postoperative respiratory difficulties so you should try to do these exercises several times a day as well.

1. **Diaphragmatic breathing.** While lying flat on your back, place your hands or a pillow over your incision. Take a series of deep breaths so that your entire abdomen, not just your lungs, expands. Repeat 6 to 8 times.

2. **Lower chest expansion.** Rest your hands on the lower part of your rib cage. Take a deep breath, and focus on trying to expand your lungs under your hands. Repeat 6 to 8 times.

3. **Upper chest expansion.** Rest your hands on the upper part of your rib cage. Take a deep breath, and focus on trying to expand your lungs under your hands. Repeat 6 to 8 times.

If your healthcare provider approves and if you're feeling strong enough to increase your daily routine, the following exercises can help you get back on the road to fitness. Add the exercises in the order shown as directed. For example, on Days 4 to 6 you will do Kegels, Breathing, Drawing In, and Clock Circles. Days 7 to 13 you will add Head Lifts and Leg Slides, and so on. After two weeks you should be able to do all of the exercises listed here every day until your postpartum checkup, at which point you can progress to the more challenging workout in the following chapter. These exercises (and the ones in Chapter 10) are courtesy of Debi Pillarella, MEd, a pre- and postnatal exercise expert based in Munster, Ind.

Days 4 to 6 after Delivery

You may still be in the hospital four days after your Cesarean, but there are a few exercises you can do in bed. Once you get home, continue with the breathing and Kegels, and incorporate the following exercises:

1. **Drawing In (for the abdominal muscles)**

    Lie on your back in bed with your knees bent, feet flat and shoulder-width apart. Take a deep breath, expanding the abdomen. Exhale; as your abdomen falls, draw your navel toward your spine. (Imagine that you're trying to get into a pair of prepregnancy jeans.) Hold the "drawn in" contraction of the abdominal wall for 10–20 seconds. Breathe normally while maintaining the contraction. Rest. Repeat 5–10 times, resting in between exercises. Progress to the point where you can eliminate the rest and complete 5–10 exercises in a row.

2. **Clock Circles** (for the thighs, abdominals, and lower back)

While in bed, lie on your back, knees slightly bent. (If you feel strain in your back with your legs extended, place a rolled up towel or pillow under your knees). Imagine your pelvis is the hands on a clock. Beginning at the 12 o'clock position, slowly lift your hips off the floor and rotate them in a clockwise position, completing one full rotation of the clock. (Be careful not to arch your back.) Rest, then reverse the direction. Repeat 3–4 clock circles in each direction. Progress to the point where you can eliminate the rest and complete 3–4 clock circles in each direction.

Days 7 to 13 after delivery

1. **Head Lifts** (for the abdominals)

If you can comfortably lie down on the floor, do this move from the floor. If it's too painful, you can do it while in bed. Lie on your back with your knees bent, shoulder-width apart and feet flat. Cross your hands over your abdomen as you cradle your belly and support your abdominal region.

Take a deep breath, expanding your abdomen and feel your belly press into your hands. Exhale. As your abdomen falls, draw your navel toward your spine. (Use that prepregnancy jeans image again.) Hold the "drawn in" contraction of your abdominal wall while slowly lifting your head off the floor. Inhale as you lower your head back to the starting position. Rest for 3–5 seconds. Repeat 5–10 times. Progress to the point where you can eliminate the rest, completing ten head lifts in a row.

2. **Leg Slides** (for the abdominals, buttocks, and legs). See Figure 5.

If you can comfortably lie down on the floor, do this move from the floor. If it's too painful, you can do it while in bed.

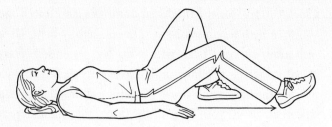

Figure 5. Leg slides.

Lie on your back with one leg extended and one leg bent, so that your foot is flat on the floor. Draw your navel toward your spine and hold firm while breathing normally. Slide the bent leg out so it is fully extended (or as far as it is comfortable) and slide it back to the bent starting position. Rest. Repeat 5–10 times before repeating with the other leg. Progress to the point where you can eliminate the rest, completing 5–10 repetitions with each leg.

Day 14 and Beyond
FIRST, CHECK FOR "DIASTASIS"

During your pregnancy your may have heard about a condition called *diastasis*. It is a separation of the two halves of the rectus abdominis muscle, the muscle that runs down the middle of your belly. To check for diastasis, lie down on your back with your knees bent. Place your fingertips one to two inches below your navel with your fingers pointing downward toward your feet. Slowly lift your head as high as possible. See if you feel a ridge protruding from the midline of your abdomen. That ridge is diastasis. If you have diastasis, be very careful not to increase the separation when doing abdominal exercises. You should cradle your abdomen with your hands (one hand on each side of the abdomen), holding the abdominis muscle together. Your range of motion should be modified so that you only raise and lower your head and don't lift your shoulders during the exercises listed below. With time, the diastasis should resolve and then you can progress into fuller range of motion exercises.

1. **Partial Curl Up (for the abdominals)**

   Lie on your back on a mat. Bend your knees so your feet are flat on the floor, shoulder-width apart. Draw your navel toward your spine and breathe normally. Extend your arms to your sides. Keeping your head in neutral alignment (chin not jutting forward or touching chest), exhale as you contract the abdominals, bringing your rib cage toward your hips, which causes your head, shoulders, and upper back to lift (approximately 45 degrees). Hold for 3–5 seconds while breathing normally. On your next inhalation, slowly lower yourself to the starting position. Rest between repetitions. Work your way up to 10–15 repetitions.

2. **Touch Downs (for the abdominals and lower back)**

   Lie on your back on a mat or soft surface. Bring both knees toward your chest. Keep your heels down toward your buttocks. Extend your arms to your sides. Keep your head in neutral alignment, with your ears in line with your shoulders. Exhale as you lift your head. Inhale and hold your head in place. Exhale and slowly lower your right bent leg so your toes touch the floor (close to your buttocks). The left bent leg remains still. Inhale as you bring your right bent leg to the starting position. Exhale as you lower your head back to the floor. Rest and repeat with the opposite leg. Work your way up to 10–15 repetitions. (Note: 1 repetition = 1 complete cycle of right leg/left leg touchdown.)

3. **Pelvic Rolling (for the hips and back)**

   Lie on your back. Bend your knees so they are side by side and your feet are flat on the floor. With your feet and shoulders on the floor, extend your arms comfortably out to the sides. While keeping your knees together and feet in their place, slowly roll your legs to the right as you turn your head toward the left. Go only as far as is comfortable for you.

Hold for 3–5 five seconds and repeat by rolling to the left and turning your head toward the right. Keep your shoulders in contact with the floor at all times. Progress to the point where you can roll your hips smoothly from side to side without resting in between. (For an exercise routine you can begin at six weeks, read Chapter 10, "The Ultimate Post–C-Section Workout.")

Diet Dos and Don'ts

At a recent health-and-fitness conference, we heard an obesity expert say that weight loss is 20 percent exercise and 80 percent nutrition. Some experts might quibble with those percentages, but the point is that the only way to lose weight—and to maintain the loss—is by watching what you eat and exercising consistently.

Start with the exercise plan above, and follow up with the exercise prescription in the next chapter and you'll be off to a great start. Then there's the other essential ingredient in the recipe for weight loss: food. When your baby becomes a toddler and starts to eat "real" food, you will be so careful about what you feed your child and be more aware than ever of your own nutritional weaknesses. Do you eat too much sugar? Skip meals? Rely on easy-to-prepare starchy carbohydrates for the bulk of your calories? Eat when you're not hungry?

Eating sensibly is always easier said than done, especially when you have a new baby to care for. But if you want to lose pregnancy weight, there's no time like the present to start. Making sure your diet consists mostly of healthy foods (complex carbohydrates like whole grains; fruits and vegetables; and lean sources of protein, such as chicken and fish) is the simplest and most sensible way to approach eating. (And if you're nursing, a healthy diet is essential!) If you're already eating this way, in order to lose weight, you simply need to trim portion sizes accordingly.

When considering dietary needs, there are some special considerations for c-section patients. Blood loss following pregnancy and surgery, as well as breast-feeding, all increase your risk for experiencing iron-deficiency or iron-deficiency anemia. According to the U.S. National Institutes of Health, iron-deficiency and iron-deficiency anemia (low levels of red blood cells due to lack of iron) are particularly common in women of childbearing age. Iron deficiency can cause a host of symptoms, including fatigue, irritability, and headaches. (And for future pregnancies, be aware that iron deficiency is linked with premature births and low-birthweight babies.) The best foods to help you boost your iron stores are leafy green vegetables, wheat germ, poultry, fish, lean red meat, dried fruit, and fortified cereals. Many of these foods are also good for digestion—and following surgery you may need all the help you can get—so they are helpful on a number of fronts. If you can squeeze it into your budget, invest in a few consultations with a registered dietician (see "Resources" for tips on how to find one in your area) who will take your special situation into account when she creates a nutrition plan for you. Whatever your postpartum situation, a dietician will advise you as to the best foods you can eat to promote your health and recovery and your baby's health (if you're breast-feeding). She will also help you figure out what your personal dietary deficiencies are, and provide simple but nutritious recipes that will make healthful cooking easier.

In the meantime, here we look at some myths about weight loss that should help you make good choices so you can lose that "baby" weight during the months to come.

Myth #1: Skipping meals is an easy way to reduce calories and lose weight.

In fact, skipping meals will send your metabolism into a tailspin and may have a seriously detrimental affect on your weight loss efforts. Skipping meals slows your metabolism—your body won't let you starve it!—increasing the amount of calories stored as fat and decreasing the number of calories you burn. Skipping meals also causes you to be extra hungry later in the day. That, in turn, leads you to make poor food choices—grabbing handy foods like chips, candy, etc.—because your primary concern is filling your empty stomach. Eating on a regular basis maintains your metabolism and allows you to experience a slow, mild hunger, which gives you time to think about and prepare nutritious foods. Breakfast is the meal that most meal-skippers skip, so at least try to fix yourself a bowl of cereal or yogurt and a glass of orange juice. Later in the morning you'll be glad you spent the five minutes it took to do this.

Myth #2: Snacking between meals is a no-no.

In fact, you're more likely to lose weight if you *do* snack. Dieticians say that spreading out your caloric intake throughout the day into five small meals encourages your body to use up the calories immediately rather than to store them for later use. Snacking also helps prevent those feelings of overwhelming hunger that sometimes compel you to overeat or make not-so-healthy food choices. Plus, it allows you more opportunities throughout the day to make smart food choices. The best snacks contain both carbohydrates (so you have instant energy) and protein (so you feel full longer and have some reserve energy). Some ideal choices include fruit with peanut butter, yogurt, cottage cheese with fruit, graham crackers with low-fat milk, nuts, or a hard-boiled egg with whole grain toast or crackers.

Myth #3. Fatty foods fill you up—and make you feel full longer—than starchy carbs (e.g., rice, pasta, bread).

In reality, fatty foods (think potato chips, cookies, French fries, donuts, etc.) may taste great, but they actually are *less* filling, at least over the course of a few hours. Protein, because it takes the longest to digest, is the food that will offer the longest feeling of fullness, next are complex carbohydrates (e.g., oatmeal or carbohydrates that come from whole grains), fat, and finally, simple carbohydrates (e.g., pastries and bread). If you eat a doughnut or muffin for breakfast, you'll probably be hungry again within an hour. But if you eat the same quantity of food, in the form of an egg or some whole grain toast and fruit, you should be able to make it to lunch without any grumbling from your tummy. One dietician we talked to explained the vicious cycle of simple carbohydrates like this: typically after eating simple carbs, we become hungry soon after and crave *more* simple carbs—it's a cycle that causes us to eat more than we need, making it very difficult to lose weight.

Myth #4: Caving into cravings will sabotage your weight-loss efforts.

You've heard the saying "The three most important words in real estate are location, location, location?" Well, the three most important words in weight loss are moderation, moderation, moderation. Ever notice how the more you try to deny yourself something, the more focused on it you become. It's the same thing with food. If you try to cut out a food that you really enjoy you'll end up giving in to your craving with gusto and maybe overindulging. If you can allow yourself special foods on occasion, though, you won't feel like you're missing out on something you love. (We can't imagine life without chocolate either!) Here's a little trick: if you love ice cream, don't keep it in the house. When you really want some, even if it's once or twice a week, make a special trip to the ice cream store and get a scoop. Rather than putting certain favorite foods on your "forbidden" list, find ways to fit them in and you'll crave them less often. Another thing to keep in mind: eating small meals throughout the day can help cut down cravings—being over-hungry increases your chances of having cravings.

Myth #5: The only equation for weight loss is calories in vs calories out.

Yes, those are two essential components of weight loss, but the third is something that's beyond your control: genetics. Some people gain—and lose—weight more easily than others. That said, know that improving your diet will lead to some weight loss and regular physical activity will, too. Continuing to exercise after you've met your weight loss goals is also the best way to keep the weight off.

How much is enough?

"My first question after my Cesarean was, 'What is the bare minimum I can eat and not compromise my healing or my milk production?' In my past pregnancies, I used pregnancy and breast-feeding as excuses to overeat and losing weight was really hard for me. This time I'm trying to eat until I feel satisfied rather than until I feel full and I'm doing a lot better, in terms of weight loss, than I did after my three vaginal births. I also realize the older I get, the more essential exercise is to weight loss and weight maintenance."

—Julie, mother of four, one Cesarean in 2003

Let's Talk About Sex . . . After Baby

With a new baby to care for 24/7, not to mention the toll that recovering from surgery takes, sex is likely to be the last thing on your mind. Understandably so. You're physically exhausted, sore, and may be feeling more emotionally overwhelmed than you'd imagined. The day will come when you and your partner are ready to resume your intimate life together. Really!

During the first few weeks, good communication is more crucial than ever because you and your baby's father are in such different physical conditions. Yes, you're both sleep deprived and worried that you're not doing everything "right," but *you* also have to heal. "This period is a test of the male partner's ability to recognize the woman's situation," Lisa Douglass, PhD, an anthropologist and expert on human sexuality, told us. "The man who is able to empathize with the new mother during this time is the one who will enjoy an enriched and deeper sexual relationship in the long run." Wondering what to expect? Here are answers to some pressing questions.

• **When is it normal to resume sex after giving birth?**

According to a recent study sponsored by the National Institute of Mental Health, 90 percent of couples have engaged in sexual intercourse within a year postpartum. Don't let that statistic alarm you! On average, couples resumed intercourse seven weeks postpartum. Women who had c-sections resumed intercourse slightly sooner than those who'd given birth vaginally. That makes sense when you consider that a Cesarean delivery doesn't leave you with the same sensitivity as a woman who delivers vaginally. Of course your surgical incision may make traditional sexual positions uncomfortable for a while, but Douglass says this is the perfect time to engage in manual or oral sex—or anything that doesn't pull at the incision or involve having the man on top. "This may be a boon to woman-oriented pleasure," she says.

Believe it or not, some women have sexual urges immediately after delivery. This may be because the body is stimulated in so many ways, and blood is drawn to the pelvic region, which increases feelings of arousal. More realistically, it will be many weeks, or even longer, before you're ready to just do it again. (Most healthcare providers recommend waiting to have intercourse until there has been no bleeding for two weeks.)

- **I want affection, but not sex—is there something wrong with me?**

No. Remember every birth is different and every postpartum period is, too. You may have wanted sex within days or weeks of delivery, or you may be happy to wait it out for months. It's important to remember, however, that sex doesn't just mean intercourse. This is a great time to expand your sexual repertoire to be more sensual, including affectionate touch, intimate conversation, massage, and so on.

You might also use this time to experiment with making your needs known, especially if you've had trouble with that in the past. Saying things like "I love it when you stroke my hair, or when we hold hands and kiss while we're watching television," will let your partner know that you appreciate his touch outside of lovemaking. If he knows that a kiss on the back of your neck while you're tending to your baby sends shivers (the good kind) down your spine, that can only be a positive thing.

"Let go of the notion that you have to get back to penetrative or 'real' sex ASAP," says Douglass. "This is a time that you can use to get to know each other all over again." In a way, of course, you are. You're getting to know each other as parents. You may even find that childbirth has made you feel more powerful and you're willing to take the lead when it comes to sex.

- **Can I please my partner even though I'm not quite up for intercourse?**

  Yes! Now is the perfect time to reexplore "manual" sex. Think back to the time when you did everything *but* intercourse. It was exciting then, and it can be just as fun now. Touching each other intimately gives you time to heal from giving birth, but the orgasms from this kind of stimulation might also help you feel like a sexual being again. This way, sex contributes rather than takes away from your healing and health. "The orgasms may even give you both the extra energy you need for those first grueling, wonderful months of a new baby's life," Douglass says. You may find that it helps to have a couple of "exploratory" and creative sessions to help you feel ready for intercourse again.

- **I think I'm ready for sex—but I'm worried about the pain, and what if my breasts leak?**

  When you think the moment is right, go for it. But take it easy. Choose a quiet time, ideally after you've fed your baby and he's likely to sleep for at least an hour so you don't feel like you have to rush through intercourse. Using a lubricant should reduce some discomfort from vaginal dryness that is expected during the postpartum period and from breast-feeding. Make sure you let your partner know what feels good and what doesn't.

  If you're breast-feeding, you may worry that your breasts will leak at an inconvenient time. And they may. During climax, some women discover that they experience let down, and their breasts spray milk. That's because the hormones that are present during orgasm are also present during let down. There's really nothing you can do about it, though the reflex does usually lessen as breast-feeding becomes more established. Just keep a towel nearby and remember that this, too, will pass. With time, sex will be as satisfying—

if not more—as it was prebaby. Sometimes tender, sometimes passionate, sometimes funny.

Scar Care

First the bad news; you will always bear some evidence of your Cesarean surgery. (Think of it as your personal badge of courage.) The scar will fade with time—and eventually be nearly invisible—but during the first few weeks and months, it will be quite red and may be swollen for the first six weeks.

Okay, so you will always see your scar. But will the area always be painful? Not exactly. The pain around your incision should subside after about six weeks. You may however, continue to feel a sensation of tugging or tension when you move in certain directions, or lift heavy objects. That we can help you do something about. In physical therapy it is quite common for physical therapists to massage a scar site to help break up the adhesions—scar tissue—that form under the skin because the adhesions can affect range of motion. "Why not do the same thing for Cesarean's scars?" asks Lynn Millar, PhD, a physical therapist and professor of physical therapy at Andrews University in Berrien Springs, Mich. "It's usual practice following Cesarean deliveries in Australia," she says.

Millar advises starting three weeks after surgery, once the incision site is healed. Take a dollop of cocoa butter or a dab of vitamin E oil and smooth it over your scar. Rub in small circular movements, about an inch of your scar at a time for about five minutes a day. If you do this regularly for a few months, it can help prevent the "tension" or pulling sensation in the lower abdomen that some women experience following a Cesarean delivery.

CHAPTER 10

The Ultimate
Post–C-Section Workout

O nce you've seen your obstetrician for your six-week postpartum visit—when you'll be checked to make sure you're healing as expected—you should be given the green light to start exercising again. Let your OB know if you plan to do an activity more strenuous than walking. If you had a complicated delivery—if you lost a lot of blood, for instance—your physician may recommend a very gradual return to exercise.

If it's "all systems go" with regard to exercise, then do we have a workout plan just for you! The Ultimate Post–C-Section Workout—designed by Debi Pillarella, MEd, a pre- and post-natal exercise expert and program manager of The Community Hospital Fitness Pointe in Munster, Ind.—combines four essential ingredients for total body fitness: aerobic activity, core toning, overall muscle strengthening, and stretching. Pillarella knows a thing or two about c-sections, having delivered both of her children this way. And she knows firsthand how tough (but not impossible) it can be to get back in shape after the surgery.

An Overview of the Four Essential Components

- **Aerobic Activity.** You will want to do some form of aerobic exercise on a regular basis—ideally on most days of the week. This is especially important if one of your goals is weight loss.

- **Core Strengthening.** "Core" is fitness lingo for the muscles of the torso. Your abdominal and back muscles did a wonderful job of supporting your baby during pregnancy. But the abuse they endured during pregnancy and from the surgery mean these muscles deserve some special attention.
- **Muscle Strengthening.** Increasing your overall muscle mass will also help you shed pregnancy weight because muscle tissue burns more calories than fat—even at rest. (Extra muscle also comes in handy for lugging all that baby gear around!)
- **Stretching.** This is the final component of the workout. If your muscles and ligaments aren't flexible, then you set yourself up for injury. Staying limber will help you enjoy your soon-to-be fit body.

Finding Time to Exercise!

One of the first challenges you'll face is finding the time to fit in exercise. There is no one schedule that works for everyone, and you may have days when you can't even find ten minutes to stretch. But if you try to do some of your exercise during one of your baby's naps, you may find that the activity refreshes you more than a nap would. And keep this in mind: some activity is always better than none. We both loved taking walks with our babies, pushing them in strollers or joggers (or carrying them in front-or backpacks). A stroller walk might not be as invigorating as a step class, but it *is* activity.

The Ultimate Workout

Equipment

Some of the exercises included in this plan require basic strength-training equipment, all of which is available at stores like Target and Wal-Mart. For about $50 you can set up a basic home gym. You'll need:

- **An exercise ball.** An oversized inflatable ball is a wonderful, versatile training tool that can be used for flexibility, strength, and balance training. Expect to pay about $20 for one.
- **Dumbbells.** To start, buy two- and five-pound weights. As you get stronger, you can add to your collection. A great option is a set of adjustable dumbbells. These usually come with several weight "plates" that allow you to add and subtract weight depending on the exercises you're doing. Dumbbells run $5 to $10 a pair, depending on the weight.
- **Resistance band.** Used for both flexibility and strength training, these bands cost about $5 and come in several different resistance levels. For starters, buy the band that has the least tension.

Choose Your Exercise Category Level

All of the exercises in this program are categorized by intensity level. Selecting a level that suits you is pretty simple: **Level 1** is your starting point. After you receive your physician's approval to begin an exercise program, begin here. Move on to **Level 2** once you can comfortably complete the Level 1 exercises. (We define, below.) When Level 2 no longer feels challenging and you're ready for a higher-intensity workout, move on to the **Challenge Level.**

The Warm-Up

Please get your healthcare provider's approval before starting a workout program. Remember, before you begin any sort of vigorous exercise, it's essential to warm up. A quick warm-up helps prepare muscles for a workout and increases blood flow. Perhaps most important, warming up is thought to reduce the risk of exercise-induced injury because it improves the flexibility in ligaments and muscles, and improves the range of motion in certain joints. A warm-up is simply five to ten minutes of a low-intensity activity, e.g., walking or marching in place, or riding a stationary bicycle slowly.

Part I. Aerobic Exercise

Always begin with a 5–10 minute warm-up and finish with a 5–minute cool-down.

1. **Level 1**—low intensity. Begin by walking at a comfortable, rhythmical pace for up to 20 minutes. If 20 continuous minutes is difficult, take two 10-minute walks. Work up to 3 times per week. Progress to Level 2 when you can complete 20 continuous minutes of aerobic exercise, 3 times per week.

2. **Level 2**—moderate intensity. Choose an enjoyable aerobic activity (bike riding, walking, jogging, swimming, etc.) that you can do for up to 30 continuous minutes, 3 to 4 times per week. Progress to the Challenge Level when you can complete the above.

3. **Challenge Level**—moderate to high intensity. Choose an aerobic activity that you can enjoy for up to 60 minutes (for low to moderate steady-paced intensity activities) or 30–45 minutes of interval (moderate to high) intensity activities, 4 to 5 times per week. An example of high-intensity intervals would be 3 minutes of walking interspersed with one minute of jogging or running.

Exercise Cautions

During exercise, if you reach a point of breathlessness, or are unable to talk, decrease your intensity. If any of the following symptoms occur during exercise, stop and contact your health care provider immediately:

• chest pain

- nausea
- severe headache or blurred vision
- unusual shortness of breath
- extremely rapid pulse that does not return to resting once intensity has been decreased
- incision pain
- any other unusual or abnormal symptoms

Part II: Core Strengthening

The core is literally your center, the place from where all movement begins. These moves are important because they will make everyday activities—especially your main one, carrying your baby—safer and more comfortable. This series is essential if you want to reshape your middle, regain strength in your back and your abdominal muscles, and ultimately banish lower back pain. These exercises target the abdominal, hip, and lower back muscles to increase muscular strength and endurance (which is why you hold some of them for what seems like a very long time!) and to improve allover balance and stability.

Do this series every day. If you are doing the core workout after your cardio workout, you do not need to warm up first. If, however, you are doing this series on a day that you are not doing an aerobic activity first, please warm up first. (See above for suggestions.)

Head/Shoulder Curl Ups (Figure 6)

LEVEL 1

a. Lie on your back with your knees bent and feet flat on the floor. (You may lie on a firm exercise mat for more comfort.) Cross your hands over your abdomen so your hands are "cradling" the abdominal area.

b. Inhale and draw your navel in (contracting abdominal mus-

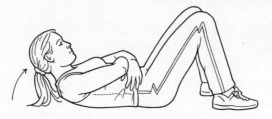

Figure 6. Head/Shoulder Curl Up.

cles) toward your spine. Exhale and lift your head (holding for 3–5 seconds), keeping your chin and neck muscles relaxed. Imagine you're holding a lemon under your chin to avoid the tendency to jut your chin forward and out of alignment. Repeat 8–10 times.

LEVEL 2

Increase to 2 sets of 10 repetitions.

CHALLENGE LEVEL

a. Add the exercise ball. Sit on the ball, feet wide apart on the floor to limit wobbling. Walk your feet out in front of you so you are lying against the ball, the small of your back comfortably pressed into the ball. Make sure your knees are bent, ankles directly beneath your knees. Your hips should be a comfortable distance apart. (Opening the hips wider will increase the stability of the exercise. Putting your knees together will decrease your stability.) Press your tongue to the roof of the mouth to prevent straining your neck muscles. Relax your head, neck, and shoulder muscles. Cross your hands over your chest.

b. While drawing your navel in toward your spine, lift your head, neck, and shoulders and lift your upper/middle back off the ball. Hold for 3–5 counts, then slowly return to starting position. Exhale on the lifting phase. Repeat 10 times, work up to 2 sets.

Alternate arm/leg reach, aka "bird dogs" (See Figure 7)

LEVEL 1

a. Kneel on all fours with your wrists directly under your shoulders, knees directly under your hips (approximately hip-width apart), and your head a natural extension of your spine (not up nor down). Your body should form a straight line from the tip of your head to the base of your tailbone.

b. Exhale and draw your navel to your spine without moving your torso. Inhale as you extend your right arm in front of you. Keep your eyes focused on the floor beneath you. Hold for 3–5 seconds, breathing normally, then slowly return to starting position on all fours. Do this exercise slowly. Don't let momentum do the work for you. Repeat the exercise on the opposite arm. Then complete the same exercise with each leg. Complete 8–10 repetitions for each arm and leg.

LEVEL 2

Start from the same position as in Level 1, but lift the opposite arm and leg simultaneously (right arm/left leg) in a slow and controlled manner. Hold for 3–5 seconds, breathing normally, then slowly return to starting position. Complete 10 repetitions on each side.

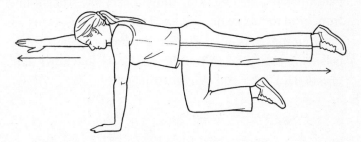

Figure 7. Alternate Arm/Leg Reach.

CHALLENGE LEVEL

Same movement as Level 2, but hold a light dumbbell or a can of soup in the "lifting" hand. For a greater challenge, add a light ankle weight (2.5 lb.) on the lifting ankle. Complete 10 repetitions on each side.

Forearm Plank (See Figure 8)

LEVEL 1

a. Kneel with your forearms on the floor; elbows directly below your shoulders and your hands clasped together. Your knees and feet should be hip-width apart and placed directly behind your hips, resting on the floor. Your head and neck should be a natural extension of your spine (do not look up or down).

b. Contract your abdominal muscles by drawing your navel to your spine. Breathe normally while holding this contraction for 30 seconds. Focus on not moving any part of your body during the hold. (The goal is to keep your body in one straight line and your abdominals contracted with normal breathing the entire time. If 30 seconds feels too long, start with 10 seconds and increase in 10-second increments until you can accomplish 30 seconds uninterrupted.) Relax and repeat 8–10 times.

LEVEL 2

Do the same move described in Level 1, but extend both legs behind you so you are balancing on your forearms and the balls of your feet. Your body should form one straight line from head to heels while you hold for 30 seconds. Don't allow your hips to bend or your back to arch. (Imagine you're balancing your baby on your hips and back and don't want him to fall.) Relax and repeat 10 times.

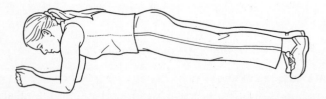

Figure 8. Forearm Plank.

CHALLENGE LEVEL

Do the same move described in Level 2, but place your forearms on a stability ball. Complete 10 repetitions. If this gets too easy, try it with your eyes closed!

Bridging (Figure 9)

LEVEL 1

a. Lie face up on the floor, feet flat on the floor, knees hip-width apart, arms relaxed at your sides, palms facing upward.

b. Contract your abdominals by drawing your navel in toward your spine while exhaling. Inhale and lift your hips until your upper torso forms a straight line from your hips to your knees. Hold for 3–5 seconds. Return to the starting position, lowering your buttocks, hips, and lower back to starting position. Complete 8–10 repetitions.

   Note: If you experience discomfort while attempting to lift your hips, to align torso, lower your hips so you are in a pain-free position. Pay attention to your alignment and avoid extreme arching of your back.

LEVEL 2

Do the same move described in Level 1, but with your bare feet on a stability ball. Complete 10 repetitions.

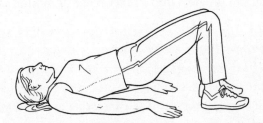

Figure 9. Bridging.

CHALLENGE LEVEL

Do the same move described in Level 2, but while using your abdominals to maintain your lifted hips, draw one knee in toward your chest. Hold for 5 seconds while taking slow deep breaths before returning to the starting position. Focus on keeping your body still and hips level while your leg is lifted. Repeat the exercise with the opposite leg. Work up to 4 sets of 10 repetitions.

Diagnosing "Diastasis"

During your pregnancy, you may have heard about a condition called diastasis. It is a separation of the two halves of the rectus abdominis muscle that runs down the middle of your belly. To check for diastasis, lie down on your back with your knees bent. Place your fingertips one to two inches below your navel with your fingers pointing downward toward your feet. Slowly lift your head as high as possible. See if you feel a ridge protruding from the midline of your abdomen. That ridge is diastasis. If you have diastasis, be very careful not to increase the separation when doing abdominal exercises. You should cradle your abdomen with your hands (one hand on each side of the abdomen), holding the abdominis muscle together. Your range of motion should be modified so that you only raise and lower your head and don't lift your shoulders during the exercises listed below. With time, the diastasis should resolve and then you can progress into a fuller range of motion exercises.

Make Proper Posture a Priority

After your Cesarean delivery, you may find yourself leaning forward while both standing and sitting. It's a subconscious reaction to the surgery, as if you are trying to protect your abdomen. Once you start carrying your baby around, this forward lean tends to increase even more because of the weight of your baby. To keep your back healthy and pressure off your abdomen, keep the following posture pointers in mind as you move through your day:

- **Keep your spine aligned.** Your ears should be directly above your shoulders; shoulders back and in alignment with your hips; your abdominal muscles drawn in, allowing your spine to be in its naturally aligned (neutral) position. Finally, don't lock your knees because this strains your back.

  Initially, avoid sitting on soft chairs and sofas because they can require extreme effort to get up from, which may hurt your incision. Soft chairs also don't usually provide much support to your back. Instead, sit in a firm, straight-backed chair. When sitting, don't slouch or arch your lower back. Placing a cushion behind your lower back can provide extra support.

- **Rise and shine slowly.** When getting out of bed, slowly roll over to one side, and then swing your legs over the edge of the bed, one at a time. Place your hands on the bed, and using the muscles of your arms, push yourself up to a sitting position.

- **Take it easy on the stairs.** Move slowly and keep your back in neutral as described above so your body weight is over your feet. Use your thigh and hip muscles to step.

- **Hold your baby (the groceries, laundry basket) close.** When reaching down to pick up an object, be sure to bend your knees and lower toward the object instead of bending from the waist. When you lift your baby or any other object, such as a bag of groceries, keep it close to your body.

- **Don't overreach.** If you need to reach something overhead, step up onto a stool. Overreaching can strain your abdominal area.

Part III: Muscle Strengthening

Motherhood requires muscle! And the muscles you need most are . . . all of them. The Core series in Part II will build strength in your abs and back, so that leaves your arms, legs, hips, and glutes (aka your butt). The combination of pregnancy and your Cesarean delivery may have caused you to use your body in awkward ways. For that reason, "functional" exercises, ones that mimic movements you do in everyday life, are the best place to start because they require you to use several muscle groups at one time . . . just as you do in everyday life. These kinds of exercises will basically train, or retrain, your large muscles to function in the right way.

> "After my c-section I thought I'd need to worry about how the incision would look, but the reality is that you can't even see the scar thanks to the pouch of fat that hangs over it! I'm back to my pre-pregnancy weight, but almost two years later I've still got the flabby stomach thing going on. The worst is when you bend over while blow-drying your hair and you see it just hanging there!"
>
> —Alicia, mother of one, c-section in 2001

As you embark on this strength-building routine, please pay close attention to how your body responds. A tingling sensation indicates that you're working the muscle to the point of fatigue. The best way to progress is to work to fatigue but not beyond. Do each of these eight moves 2–3 times per week but always with at least one day of rest in between. The Level 1 workout will take about 20 minutes, the Challenge Level about 30. Of course, you don't have to do all eight moves at once, either. You can do half in the morning and half in the evening or whatever best fits your schedule.

Lunges (strengthen hips, thighs, and buttocks). See Figure 10.
LEVEL 1

a. Stand with proper posture (described in "Make Proper Posture a Priority"). Place your hands on your hips, or let them relax at your side, and take one step forward so one foot is in front of the other. The distance between the two feet should be approximately one stride length. The hips should be squared so both hip bones are facing forward. Draw the navel in toward the spine.

b. Stay erect and bend your knees so your torso lowers to the point where your front thigh is parallel to the ground. Keep your navel drawn back toward your spine. Your front knee should be directly above your front heel. Do not let your knees drift forward over your toes because this puts too much stress on the knees. Hold for 3–5 seconds, then straighten your knees so your torso returns to its starting position. Step forward with the opposite leg. Repeat 8–10 times for each leg.

LEVEL 2

Do the same move described in Level 1, but hold a light dumbbell (2–3 lb.) in each hand. Complete 10 repetitions for each leg. Work up to 2 sets.

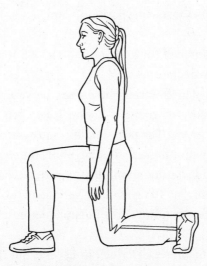

Figure 10. Lunges.

CHALLENGE LEVEL

Do the same move described in Levels 1 and 2, but step onto a stair or an aerobics step, about 6"–8" high. Complete 10 repetitions for each leg. Work up to two sets.

Squats (strengthen hips, thighs, and buttocks). See Figure 11.

LEVEL 1

a. Stand with feet hip-width apart, knees slightly bent but above your ankles. Check spine alignment: ears should be directly above shoulders, shoulders relaxed. Hold your arms straight out in front of you or let them hang at your sides.

b. Contract your abdominal muscles by drawing your navel in toward your spine. Exhale as you bend your knees, lowering your torso toward the floor. Your hips should move down and back as if you were going to sit on a chair. Your knees should remain above your ankles, not over your toes. When your thighs are parallel to the floor, hold for 3–5 seconds. Do not lean forward from your waist. Breathe normally while holding the contraction. Inhale as you slowly straighten your knees, returning to the starting position. Complete 8–10 repetitions.

LEVEL 2

a. Place a dumbbell (or a ten-pound sack of potatoes) on the floor between your legs.

b. At the end of the lowering phase grasp the weight. Hold it close to your body, imagining it is your baby, then return to the starting position. The next time you squat, return the weight to the floor. Continue alternating lifting the weight and placing it back on the floor until all the repetitions have been completed. Complete 10 repetitions, work up to two sets.

CHALLENGE LEVEL (also works the oblique muscles in the abdominal area)

Do the same move described in Level 2, but this time after you return to the starting position with the weight held

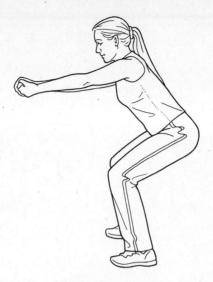

Figure 11. Squats.

close to your body, exhale and twist to one side of your body, looking over your shoulder. Repeat and on the next "weighted" lifting phase, twist to the other side of the body. Pretend you are passing your baby to his grandmother to help you keep the move slow and controlled. Complete 10 repetitions, work up to two sets.

Step Up/Lunge Back (strengthens hips, thighs, and buttocks). See Figure 12.

LEVEL 1

a. Begin facing a step (no more than 8" high). Your ears should be directly above your shoulders, shoulders relaxed. Your arms should hang to either side of your body, as a natural extension of the upper body. Draw your navel in toward your spine, relax your hips and knees. Try not to lean forward or back.

b. With your hands resting on your hips, draw your navel in toward your spine, then step up with your left foot. Keep

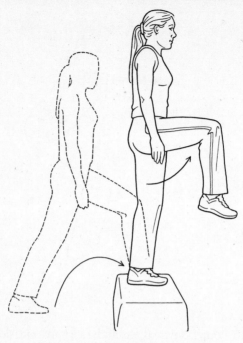

Figure 12(A). Step Up/Lunge Back.

your foot flat on top of the step while you straighten the left knee, lifting the right leg off the floor. Lift the right knee no higher than hip level. (12A) Hold for 3–5 seconds. Step down with your right foot. Step down and back with the left foot so you end up in a split lunge; both knees bent. Straighten the knees and bring the left foot back to the starting position. Keep your upper body still during this move. Take care to maintain knee-over-ankle alignment to protect your knees. (12B) Repeat, beginning with the opposite foot. Complete 8–10 repetitions for each leg.

LEVEL 2

Do the same move described in Level 1 while holding 5–10 pound dumbbells, hands at your sides. Complete 10–15 repetitions.

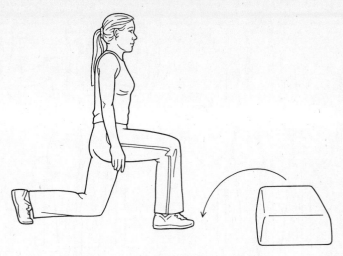

Figure 12(B). Step Up/Lunge Back.

CHALLENGE LEVEL

Do the same move described in Level 2, but work up to 2 sets.

Push-Ups (strengthens chest, shoulders, biceps, and triceps)

LEVEL 1

a. Kneel on the ground on all fours. Your head and neck should be a natural extension of your spine; your elbows relaxed; your wrists should be directly under your shoulders; your shoulders relaxed.

b. Position your knees so they are shoulder-width apart, directly under your hips; your feet and ankles should be relaxed. Draw the navel into the spine without moving the torso. Bend your elbows, lowering your chest to the floor. Hold for 3–5 seconds. Exhale as you straighten your elbows and slowly return to the starting position. Complete 8–10 repetitions.

LEVEL 2

Do the same move described in Level 1, but lower your entire torso to the floor. Work up to 10–15 repetitions.

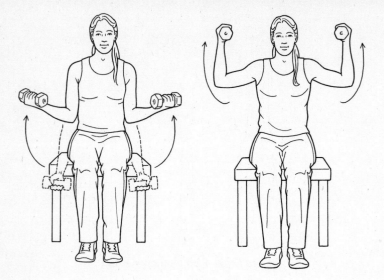

Figure 13. Curl and Lift.

CHALLENGE LEVEL

Do the same move described in Level 2, but work up to two sets. If you want to vary the move, and make it more challenging, spread your hands farther apart.

Curl and Lift (strengthens biceps and shoulders). See Figure 13.

LEVEL 1

a. Sit on the edge of an armless chair with your feet on the floor, arms hanging down naturally at your sides. Hold a dumbbell (3–5 lb.) in each hand, palms facing forward.

b. Draw your navel in toward your spine. Exhale, bend your elbows, and bring the dumbbells toward the shoulders, stopping when your elbows are at a 90-degree angle. With your elbows at your sides, lift your arms to either side, stopping when the arms are at shoulder height. The elbows remain bent. Retrace the exercise steps in the reverse order; lowering arms to your sides (elbows at your waist), then straightening your elbows, lowering your arms to the starting position position. Complete 8–10 times on each side.

LEVEL 2

Do the same move described for Level 1, but while sitting on the stability ball to add the challenge of maintaining your balance (which forces you to recruit your core muscles). Work up to two sets of 10–15 repetitions.

CHALLENGE LEVEL

Do the same move described in Level 2 but increase the weight slightly. Work up to two sets of 10–15 repetitions.

Seated Row (strengthens upper back). See Figure 14.

LEVEL 1

a. Using a light to moderate resistance band, place the band around the leg of a sturdy piece of furniture (e.g., a table, a couch or recliner chair). Sit on the floor, facing the furniture with your knees bent and legs extended. Grasp the handles of the band (one handle in each hand) so your

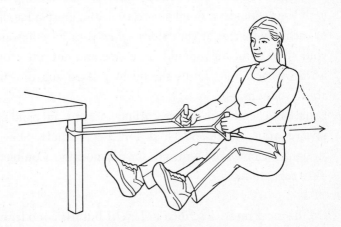

Figure 14. Seated Row.

arms are extended in front of you. Draw your navel toward your spine.

b. Keeping your shoulders down and navel drawn in, contract your upper shoulder blade muscles as if trying to squeeze a dollar bill between them. Bend your elbows as you pull the resistance band back. Hold for 3–5 seconds. Straighten your elbows as you slowly bring your arms back to the starting position. Keep your torso still for the duration of the move. Complete 8–10 repetitions.

LEVEL 2

Do the same move described in Level 1, but increase repetitions to 15.

CHALLENGE LEVEL

Do the same move described in Levels 1 and 2, but work up to two sets of 10–15 repetitions.

Biceps Curl (strengthens biceps). See Figure 15.

LEVEL 1

a. Stand on top of your resistance band, feet shoulder-width apart, knees slightly bent. Make sure your ears are aligned with your shoulders, shoulders relaxed, and grasp a handle in each hand, arms at your sides. Draw your navel toward your spine. Your hips should be relaxed and not tilted forward or back. Your knees should be relaxed and directly above your ankles.

b. Exhale and bend your elbows, curling the arms and band up toward your shoulders. Hold for 3–5 seconds. Slowly straighten elbows and return to starting position. Complete 8–10 repetitions.

LEVEL 2

Do the same move described in Level 1 but use a moderate dumbbell (5–10 pounds) instead of the band. Complete 10–15 repetitions.

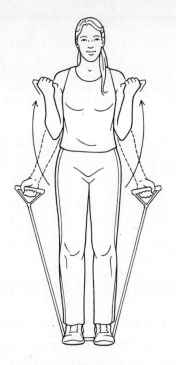

Figure 15. Biceps Curl.

CHALLENGE LEVEL

Do the same move described in Levels 1 and 2, but while sitting on a stability ball. Work up to two sets of 10 repetitions.

Row and Kickback (strengthens biceps, triceps, and shoulders). See Figure 16.

LEVEL 1

a. Standing next to a chair, place your right knee on the seat, left foot flat on the floor.

b. Place your right hand on the arm of the chair. (16A) Bend forward so your back is parallel to the floor. Hold a light to moderate weight dumbbell (3–8 pounds) in your left hand. Your arm is extended down and directly under your shoulder. Your palm is facing in. Draw your navel in toward your spine.

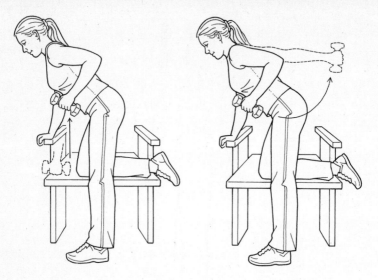

Figure (16A) In position to row. (16B) The kickback.

c. Bend your left elbow up toward the ceiling. (16B) Keep your shoulder and hips facing the floor. Hold for 3–5 seconds. Straighten your elbow, pressing the dumbbell behind you. Bend the elbow back to where it came from. Straighten the elbow so you are back to starting position. Keep the movement slow and controlled so you don't allow momentum to do the work for you. Complete 8–10 repetitions on one side and then repeat with the other side.

LEVEL 2

Do the same move described in Level 1 but increase repetitions to 10–15 for each side.

CHALLENGE LEVEL

Do the same move described in Level 2 but work up to two sets of 8–10 repetitions.

The Cool-Down

Cooling down after exercise helps lower your body temperature and can reduce muscle soreness. A cool-down should be approximately five minutes in length and can include the same kinds of low intensity activities you did for the warm-up. Then finish with the series of stretches that follow. Since "cold" muscles are more prone to injury, it's always safer to stretch at the end of a workout (or after a short warm-up).

Part IV: Stretching

In addition to your cardiovascular and strengthening exercises, it's imperative that you include daily stretching. The following two stretch sequences are designed to not only stretch the muscles you've worked, but also to enhance your overall range of motion, especially in the area of your incision. Remember that stretching should feel rejuvenating, and never painful. Your breathing should be slow, deep, and mindful. That means exhale into the stretch, allowing 3 to 4 seconds for the exhalation and inhale on the return from the stretch, allowing another 3 to 4 seconds. Take two slow deep breaths between stretches.

Level 1—Repeat each individual stretch 2–3 times with a short rest in between.

Level 2—Allow the stretches to flow into each other. Complete 1 entire sequence, then rest. Complete a second sequence, then rest.

Challenge Level—Complete the stretch sequence in a flowing manner. Complete 2 stretch sequences before resting.

. . . .

Stretch Sequence 1

Seated "C" Stretch (for the spine)

1. Sit on the floor with your knees about shoulder-width apart and your hands grasping the back of your thighs. Allow your elbows to relax at your sides. Keep your head and spine in neutral alignment; chin drawn in, looking straight ahead, shoulders, down and under your ears, navel drawn in toward your spine.

2. Exhale and tilt your pelvis and curl your body into a letter "C" position. Draw your navel in toward your spine while relaxing the muscles of the pelvic floor. Hold this position for 3–5 seconds as you slowly breathe normally. Breathe normally and slowly return to your starting position.

Butterfly/Look to the Sky (for the inner thighs)

1. Sit on the floor with your knees and ankles together, feet on the floor. Your hands should be placed on the inner part of each thigh, knuckles touching each other.
2. Exhale as you slowly open your legs, guiding them with your palms, until you get to a comfortable open hip position. Imagine your legs are wings on a butterfly opening to fly. Hold this position for 3–5 seconds as you slowly breathe normally. Place your hands on the outside of your knees as you slowly return to the starting position. When you get to the starting position, place your hands on the floor behind your buttocks, fingers pointing sideways. Press the palms of your hands into the ground as you exhale and look toward the sky. Hold this position for 3–5 seconds as you slowly breathe normally. Slowly return to your starting position.

Spinal Twist (for the spine)

1. Sit on the floor with your knees bent, and ankles touching, feet on the floor.
2. Inhale as you place your left hand across your right thigh. Exhale as you place your right hand on the floor behind your right buttock, twisting your spine and looking over your right shoulder. Hold this position for 3–5 seconds as you slowly breathe normally. Breathe normally and slowly return to your starting position. Repeat in the opposite direction.

Roll Down/Up (for the spine)

1. Sit on the floor with your knees shoulder-width apart, feet on the floor and hands under your thighs.

2. Draw your navel toward your spine. Exhale and curl your spine as you begin to roll down toward the floor. The tailbone will make contact with the floor first, followed by your low back, mid back, upper back, shoulders, neck, and finally head. Pay attention to releasing stress and tension as each body part relaxes into the floor beneath you. Once you get to a full lying position, imagine you are melting into the floor, totally relaxed. Hold this position for 3–5 seconds. Exhale, slowly reverse the action, rolling up to return to your starting position. Take 2 deep breaths before repeating. At the end of this stretch, remain flat on the floor.

Full-Body Stretch

1. Lie on the floor with your arms naturally extended at your sides, palms facing upward and legs naturally extended from your hips, feet relaxed and uncrossed.

2. Close your eyes. Inhale as you bring your arms overhead and then rest them on the floor. Reach your right leg and left arm as far apart from each other as possible, as if you are trying to add a couple of inches to your length. Hold for three to five seconds, breathing normally. Reach your left leg and right arm as far apart from each other as possible. Hold for 3 to 5 seconds, breathing normally. Reach both arms and both legs as far apart from each other as possible. Hold for 3 to 5 seconds, breathing normally. Bring arms back to the sides of your body for total relaxation. Take full "belly" breaths while keeping your eyes closed. Say "Aaaah" on each exhalation. If you're holding a lot of stress and/or tension, place your finger pads of your index and middle fingers on either temple and make small circles while deep breathing.

. . . .

Stretch Sequence 2

Cow/Cat Stretch (for the spine)

1. Kneel on all fours with your hands flat on the ground, wrists slightly in front of your shoulders and knees directly under your hips, about hip-width apart.

2. Keeping your arms straight, inhale as your head and tailbone tilt upward, creating an arch in your back (in yoga, this is referred to as the cow posture). Hold 3 to 5 seconds breathing normally. Draw your navel to your spine as you exhale and continue pressing your navel upward, letting your head and tailbone move downward, rounding your spine like a cat. Hold for 3 to 5 seconds breathing normally.

Child's Pose (for the shoulders, arms, and spine)

1. Kneel on the ground on all fours, with your wrists slightly in front of your shoulders; knees directly under hips, about hip-width apart.

2. Keeping your arms straight, exhale as you sit back onto your heels to rest. Hold 3–5 seconds and breathe normally. If sitting onto your heels causes pain in your knees, place a thick pillow between your buttocks and your heels to keep your hips elevated.

Downward Facing Dog (for the spine, shoulders, and hamstrings)

1. Kneel on the ground on all fours, your wrists slightly in front of your shoulders; knees directly under hips, about hip-width apart.

2. Exhale, pressing your body weight back, straightening your knees, and bringing the soles of your feet to the floor. Lift your hips in the air, legs straight (knees bent if needed) to form an inverted "V." Press your heels toward the floor as

your palms press away from the floor, your head hanging between your arms. Hold for 3 to 5 seconds. Walk your hands backward toward your feet, bend your knees, and prepare for "rag doll roll-up." (NOTE: Avoid this stretch if you have high blood pressure.)

Rag Doll Roll-Up / Reach to The Sky (for the hamstrings and spine)

a. Begin in ending position of "downward facing dog," where you are bent forward in a standing position, hands on floor in front of feet. (NOTE: If this is difficult, place hands atop the knees.) Bend the knees slightly.

b. Slowly roll up as if you are a "rag doll," stacking the vertebrae one at a time. Leave your arms hanging, as they will follow the progressive roll-up. Roll your shoulders back so they are under your ears. Lift your neck and head as natural extensions of your spine with your chin not extending forward or backward. Take 2 deep breaths when you get to the upright position. Inhale as you bring your arms overhead and reach toward the sky. Reach right arm higher than left. Repeat with left arm reaching higher than the right. Breathe normally and slowly return both arms to the sides of the body.

. . . .

Be patient with your body

"I have always been very active—I walked five miles the day my first child was born. So when I had to have an emergency c-section and then could barely walk from my bedroom to the bathroom for two whole weeks, it was shocking for me. I really didn't anticipate how challenging it would be to get back into shape. Within 8–12 weeks of my son's birth I was exercising, but it took me about 5–6 months before I was back to doing all my normal activities. I just wish I had known what to expect."

—Monica, mother of two, two Cesareans in 1999 and 2001

. . . .

Sample Workout Calendar – Level 1

SUNDAY	MONDAY	TUESDAY	WEDNESDAY	THURSDAY	FRIDAY	SATURDAY
	20 min. cardio		20 min. cardio		20 min. cardio	Leisure activities*
Core series	Core series	Core series	Core series	Core series	Core series	Core series
			Strength-training		Strength-training	
Stretch sequence #1	Stretch sequence #2	Stretch sequence #1	Stretch sequence #2	Stretch sequence #1	Stretch sequence #2	Stretch sequence #1

Sample Workout Calendar – Level 2

SUNDAY	MONDAY	TUESDAY	WEDNESDAY	THURSDAY	FRIDAY	SATURDAY
	up to 30 min. cardio	up to 30 min. cardio	up to 30 min. cardio		up to 30 min. cardio	Leisure activities*
Core series	Core series	Core series	Core series	Core series	Core series	Core series
			Strength-training		Strength-training	
Stretch sequence #1	Stretch sequence #2	Stretch sequence #1	Stretch sequence #2	Stretch sequence #1	Stretch sequence #2	Stretch sequence #1

Sample Workout Calendar – Challenge Level

SUNDAY	MONDAY	TUESDAY	WEDNESDAY	THURSDAY	FRIDAY	SATURDAY
	up to 60 min. cardio	up to 60 min. cardio	up to 60 min. cardio		up to 60 min. cardio	Leisure activities*
Core series	Core series	Core series	Core series	Core series	Core series	Core series
		Strength-training		Strength-training		Strength-training
Stretch sequence #1	Stretch sequence #2	Stretch sequence #1	Stretch sequence #2	Stretch sequence #1	Stretch sequence #2	Stretch sequence #1

* Leisure activities such as walking your baby in a stroller, cycling, etc.

CHAPTER 11

Future Pregnancies

As you look forward to future pregnancies, you may have questions about how your previous Cesarean will affect your ability to get pregnant. And when you do find out that you're pregnant again, we suspect one of the first questions you'll ask your OB is about the delivery. "Should I have another Cesarean?" "*Can* I have another Cesarean?" "Can I attempt a vaginal birth this time around?"

First, a look at some of the long-term effects that result from a c-section delivery:

- Uterine scarring from a Cesarean can affect implantation. When there's less healthy tissue available for an egg to implant, it can mean more difficulty getting pregnant.
- A 1996 Finnish study suggests that women who've had a Cesarean birth are more likely to have ectopic pregnancies than women who have not had a surgical birth.
- A previous Cesarean can increase the risk of placental problems in future pregnancies. As we mention in the first chapter, placental problems can lead to a Cesarean birth, or in this case, a repeat Cesarean. According to ACOG, women who have had at least one Cesarean delivery are 2.6 times more likely to develop placenta previa (a condition in which the placenta blocks the vaginal opening) in a future pregnancy. Other studies have shown that this risk goes up with each subsequent pregnancy.

- A previous Cesarean also increases your chances of developing placenta accreta, a life-threatening condition in which the placenta adheres to the uterine wall, making the placenta extremely difficult or impossible to remove. (This condition can't be diagnosed until the physician attempts to remove the placenta during the surgery. If there are problems removing the placenta, the patient is at risk for hemorrhage and infection due to the lengthened surgery. There's also the possibility a hysterectomy will be needed to prevent the woman from bleeding to death.) While this condition occurs in only 4.5 percent of pregnancies of women who have not had previous uterine surgery, that percentage jumps to between 24 percent and 38 percent in women who have placenta previa and have uterine scarring, including from a previous Cesarean. Some physicians believe this risk alone is a reason to try to reduce the overall rate of Cesarean births.

VBAC vs C-Peat

The decision about whether to have a repeat Cesarean or attempt a VBAC should be one that you make after careful consultation with your physician and/or midwife. When your healthcare provider offers a recommendation, she will consider your medical history, the circumstances surrounding your previous Cesarean, and the resources available to you at the hospital where you will deliver. If you insist on attempting a VBAC against your obstetrician's advice, be aware that you will probably need to look for another OB.

If you had no problems dealing with or recovering from your first Cesarean, anticipating a repeat might not be a big deal. In fact, a "c-peat," as we've dubbed it, might be your preference. But if you were disappointed by your birth experience, if you wonder if the Cesarean was really necessary, you might be more conflicted. The decision about whether to opt for another Cesarean or attempt a vaginal birth may even make you anxious about being pregnant.

In the obstetrics community, opinions about which option should be recommended are split. Within the last few years we've seen more and more obstetricians lean toward recommending a repeat Cesarean. One reason for the return to recommending a c-peat, is that beginning in the 1980s, when the percentage of women attempting a VBAC started to increase, so did the rate of both maternal and infant mortality.

While the overall risk for uterine rupture and injury or death to the baby is still very small, many physicians feel that encouraging a woman to undergo a "trial of labor" so that she can attempt a vaginal birth is simply not worth the risk. In a 2001 *New England Journal of Medicine* editorial entitled "Vaginal Delivery after Cesarean Section—Is the Risk Acceptable?" the author of the editorial, Michael F. Greene, MD, of Massachusetts General Hospital, concludes that a repeat Cesarean is safest for both mother and baby. "After a thorough discussion of the risks and benefits of attempting a vaginal delivery after Cesarean section, a patient might ask, 'But doctor, what is the safest thing for my baby?' Given the findings of [a study of 20,095 women], my unequivocal answer is: elective repeated Cesarean section."

If a woman's uterus does rupture during labor, the risk of infant death increases tenfold. Another motivating factor for recommending a repeat c-section, may be that physicians are unwilling to risk being held liable should the VBAC have tragic results.

On the other hand, there are obstetricians and midwives who believe that the increasing Cesarean rate is simply too high and that every effort should be made to encourage women to consider a VBAC. They believe that if the VBAC is successful, a woman stands to benefit from a lower risk of postpartum infection, a shorter hospital stay, and a faster recovery. If the woman plans future pregnancies, she also has a lower risk of placental problems, such as placenta accreta, because this condition is associated with Cesarean births.

What You Need to Know About VBAC

There are entire books devoted to this topic, but for starters, if a VBAC is your goal, you will have to find a physician who is willing to help you achieve it. Because there is a small risk of uterine rupture even with the low transverse incision—this life-threatening event happens to about 1 percent of women who've had one Cesarean and are attempting VBAC—many hospitals now require, for liability's sake, that an obstetrician be "immediately" available in case a repeat is necessary. For some hospitals, especially smaller and nonteaching ones, this is cost-prohibitive. Some physicians are also unwilling to be present at a hospital for the entire duration of a patient's labor simply because she has had one c-section. They'd rather just schedule the surgery at a time that's convenient.

If you plan to attempt a VBAC, one of the best things you can do is to give your uterus enough time to adequately heal. Women whose deliveries are spaced fewer than eighteen months apart—nine months or less between pregnancies—have a greater than usual risk of uterine rupture if they've had a c-section. One study reviewed the records of more than 2,400 women who attempted labor after having had one Cesarean. Within that group there were twenty-nine uterine ruptures, a rate of 1.2 percent. But within the subgroup of women who were delivering their second baby within 18 months of having had the Cesarean, the rate of uterine rupture was nearly twice that. Still a small percentage, roughly 2.25 percent, but worth considering. The researchers theorize that it takes six months, possibly nine, for the uterus to heal completely following a Cesarean birth.

The benefits of VBAC

You've already gone through one Cesarean delivery, why consider a vaginal birth? If you're successful, you'll have a shorter hospital stay and recovery period, a lower risk of dangerous blood clots, less need for transfusion, lower risk of postpartum infection, and less risk of serious complications in future pregnancies. It's important to keep two things in mind: although some sources say that 60–80 percent of women who attempt VBAC are successful, most of the studies don't include women who are thought to be "inappropriate" candidates for trial of labor, according to ACOG. Therefore, it might be more a more accurate reflection of the statistics to state that 60–80 percent of women who meet all of the criteria to attempt a VBAC are successful. And second, neither trial of labor and VBAC nor a repeat Cesarean is risk free.

Want to try a VBAC? Can you say "Yes" to the following questions?

- **Do you have the support of your physician?** As we mentioned above, one reason physicians are hesitant to recommend a VBAC is the very real risk of malpractice suits. However, if your doctor isn't supportive of a VBAC, and there's no medical reason to warrant a repeat c-section, find another doctor who will see you through the labor. Teaching hospitals often have the highest VBAC success rate, so that's one place to start. The reason for this is teaching hospitals have resident physicians on site 24-hours a day so having a physician "immediately available" is a VBAC criterion that can be met.

- **Is your pelvis intact and adequate for a vaginal birth?** This simply means that your pelvis must be large enough to allow a baby to fit through and that you have no abnormalities or illness that might prevent a vaginal birth or make it too risky.

- **Did you have a low transverse uterine incision with your last c-section(s)?** This isn't the scar you see on your abdomen just above your pubic bone, but the one that's on your uterus. You may, in fact, have had a low transverse incision on your abdomen but a different type of incision on your uterus. If you are seeing a different physician for subsequent pregnancies, make sure you have a copy of your medical records from your previous Cesarean birth. This information will be included in your record. Unlike a vertical incision, a transverse incision is less likely to rupture during childbirth, which makes a VBAC less risky.

- **Is the hospital where you plan to deliver equipped for an emergency c-section?** If the hospital isn't able to perform an emergency c-section safely 24 hours a day, it is unlikely you will be allowed to attempt a VBAC. Nor should you labor at home with the hope that you'll get to the hospital once labor is well underway. A uterine rupture is a potentially life-threatening condition for both mother and baby. While it's uncommon, should this scenario develop, a quick Cesarean delivery is needed to protect the mother and baby.

What can you do to increase your chances of a successful VBAC?

- **Commit yourself to it.** Some experts believe that feeling confident about your decision can positively impact the outcome. Experts say that women who really desire a VBAC have a lower repeat Cesarean rate. The opposite can also be true. Several studies suggest that fear of labor can actually stop progress and increase the odds of an emergency Cesarean birth. One of the best ways to become comfortable and confident about your decision is to read up on the subject and consult reputable Web sites and groups that offer support. Two we can recommend are www.vbac.com and www.acog.org. You should also find out if your local hospital offers a VBAC class or support group for you and your partner. Having a partner who is behind your decision to try a VBAC is a plus in the labor and delivery room.

- **Tell your physician you do not want cervical ripening/labor-inducing drugs.** Using these may increase the risk of uterine rupture during a trial of labor because they can "hyperstimulate" the uterus and cause more forceful contractions than you might have without the drugs.
- **Hold off on the epidural.** Having an epidural can increase your total labor by an average of an hour. The longer your labor, the higher your chances of delivering by c-section.
- **Consider adding a midwife or doula to your labor support team.** One study suggests that the added support could reduce the odds of a Cesarean by 50 percent.

An ideal VBAC candidate

"When I went into labor with my first child, everything was going fine until he decided he was happy to stay right in the birth canal. The official diagnosis was "dystocia," and he ultimately was delivered by Cesarean. When my second child was due, about two years later, my OB recommended that I try for a vaginal birth and it was something I really wanted to do. It went very smoothly, not a single complication, and my daughter was born vaginally. I ended up having two more VBACs after that one. I don't feel that one mode of delivery is necessarily better than the other, but my recovery from the vaginal births was certainly easier than with the Cesarean."

—Lia, mother of four, one Cesarean in 1990, three VBACs

When a VBAC Won't Work

Reasons you should not consider a VBAC with your next pregnancy:

- You have a uterine scar that extends into the fundus, either from a previous classical or T-shaped Cesarean or other similar uterine surgery.
- You have a misshapen pelvis, either from a birth defect, an injury, or illness.
- You have a medical condition, including diabetes, hypertension, obesity, herpes, or HIV that makes a repeat Cesarean a safer option.
- You live in an area where emergency medical situations cannot be handled quickly. This may mean you live in a rural area where the obstetrician and anesthesiologist might not be immediately available.

VBAC at Home? Don't Do It

There has been perhaps some unexpected fallout due to many physicians' reluctance to encourage trial of labor and VBAC, and insurance companies' reluctance to allow it: women who wish to attempt a VBAC are opting for home birth. While we acknowledge that around the world billions of women have successfully given birth at home, we have just five words to say about this issue: Home deliveries are for pizza—especially when you have had a previous c-section.

FAQs When Planning a Repeat Cesarean

Q. What are the risks of a repeat Cesarean birth?

A. They are basically the same as they were with your previous Cesarean: infection, hemorrhage, injury, problems with anesthesia, all of which can be serious enough to be life-threatening. (The risk of death from a c-section is approximately 3 to 7 times greater than from a vaginal birth.) Your baby is also at higher risk of developing an upper respiratory infection if delivered by c-section.

Q. **What are the benefits of a repeat Cesarean birth?**

A. You don't have to go through labor, which, for some women is more painful and scary than the incision that follows a c-section. Also, because the baby doesn't pass through the birth canal, some studies suggest that women lessen their risk of damage to the bladder, perineum, and bowels. Research in this area is inconclusive—talk with your physician about this issue. Injury to these areas has been associated with an increased risk of urinary and fecal incontinence as well as pelvic-organ prolapse, a condition which must be fixed with surgery.

Q. **Can I schedule the Cesarean for a day that's convenient for me?**

A. More or less. If you are in a practice with one obstetrician or prefer one over another in a practice, the physician's surgery schedule will dictate which days you get to choose. If you schedule months ahead of time (hospitals often have you wait until you're in your last trimester before scheduling) you can ask for an early morning surgery, rather than wait until later in the day.

Q. **The hospital where I will deliver is very busy; how can I find out when it's the least busy?**

A. While there are definitely certain times of the year when more babies are born, it can be pretty hard to predict which day of the week has the fewest surgeries at your hospital. On average, the weekends tend to be the slowest times when you consider both vaginal and Cesarean births. But often you don't have the option of scheduling a surgery on the weekend.

Q. **What time of day is best for surgery?**

A. Morning. If you schedule your Cesarean for early morning, it is less likely that your procedure will get bumped due to unforeseen circumstances such as other emergency c-sections.

Q. What should I do to prepare for the surgery?

A. Other than scheduling it through the hospital and eating a semiliquid diet for forty-eight hours before, to help reduce postsurgery gas pains, there's not much you need to do. Since you'll know the exact date, you can arrange to have help lined up the day you come home from the hospital. Definitely treat yourself to some pre-Cesarean pampering: get a good night's sleep the day before, have a pedicure, see a matinee, lunch with your girlfriends, and have a date with your spouse!

Q. Can I expect the same thing from the surgery?

A. Pretty much. If your previous Cesarean followed labor, one thing that will be different this time is that you'll get to walk into the operating room. A repeat c-section can also take a little longer than your first since the OB will have to cut through scar tissue that may have adhered to other areas, such as the bowel. If you labored before your first c-section, you can expect your recovery time to be easier the second time around since this time you won't be exhausted from labor.

- -

My scheduled cesarean was a piece of cake

"My first Cesarean was an emergency that followed a difficult labor and it was so scary that I didn't want to risk having that experience again. So there was no question for me that I'd have a repeat. I felt absolutely no stress with the scheduled c-section. I knew what to expect, and emotionally it was very easy the second time around. I think anyone who has had an emergency Cesarean, followed by a scheduled one, feels that way."

—Monica, mother of two Cesareans in 1999 and 2001

- -

Creating a Birth Plan for a Scheduled Cesarean

During each of our first pregnancies, we both created elaborate birth plans that outlined exactly what we "wanted" to happen during labor. Of course, what we learned is that no matter how prepared you might be for labor, stuff happens. Stuff that is way beyond our control.

So, with that in mind, during our second pregnancies we were much more flexible with the process of childbirth. But that's not to say that we were willing to relinquish every element of our babies' birth days to the physicians.

We encourage you to create a birth plan because, at the very least it requires that you think about what kind of birth you'd like to have. Creating a birth plan will also help you start a dialogue with your physician about your baby's birth. In some cases hospital policy will prevent some of your requests from being met, but at least you can have a conversation about why and see if your physician can work out some compromises.

Your birth plan can be as elaborate or simple as you wish. Here is a sample of some details that you might include:

- Since a Cesarean is necessary, we request _____ that _____ and _____ be allowed into the operating room for the duration of the procedure. We understand the OR is a sterile environment and will take the necessary precautions.
- We request that _____ be allowed to cut the umbilical cord. We understand that certain precautions must be taken and are willing to take them.
- We would like the blood from our baby's cord to be preserved for potential medical needs later in his life. We have made (or will make) arrangements with the hospital regarding this issue.

- We request that if the baby is born without complications warm towels be available so that _____ be allowed to hold the baby before he is placed in a warming device.
- We want to be able to hold our baby before he is moved to the nursery.
- We want our baby to have the opportunity to try to breast-feed as soon as possible following his delivery.
- If the baby must be transferred to a special care nursery, we request that _____ be allowed to accompany him.
- We request that one of us be with our baby during all routine medical procedures.
- If our baby is a boy, we choose to circumcise him and we would like _____ to be with our baby during the circumcision.
- If our baby is a boy, we choose *not* to circumcise him.
- Our preference is for our baby to be in mom's room.
- Our preference is for exclusive breast-feeding.
- Our preference is for exclusive bottle feeding.
- Our preference is to combine breast-feeding and bottle feeding.
- We request that our baby not be given pacifiers, formula, and sugar water because we feel these may interfere with breast-feeding.
- If our baby should die during childbirth we would like a call placed to _____ and we would like the opportunity to be alone with and hold our baby.

Resource Guide

Chapter 1: Why a Cesarean?

For more information about the history of Cesarean births, visit the National Library of Medicine's online exhibition, "Cesarean Section: A Brief History," at http://www.nlm.nih.gov/exhibition/cesarean/cesarean_2.html

Chapter 2: The Surgery

If you're interested in learning even more about the anesthesia used during childbirth, the University of Chicago has a detailed Web site with information that you might find interesting. Check out http://daccx.bsd.uchicago.edu/manuals. Click on "Anesthesia for the Pregnant Patient."

Chapter 4: Your C-Section Baby (and General Children's Health Information)

http://www.aap.org is the American Academy of Pediatrics' official Web site. It has information ranging from current treatments for asthma to links to support groups for cancer patients and advocacy information. Check out "The best of the pediatric internet," at www.aap.org/bpi for links to hundreds of sites with information about children's health.

http://www.pedinfo.org is a Web site sponsored by the University of Alabama. It includes links to dozens of sites related to children's health; to date there's an index of about 1,500.

http://www.neonatology.org is a Web site designed for healthcare professionals, but you will find information about hundreds of diseases that may help you gain understanding of your child's condition.

http://www.kidshealth.org is another helpful Web site with general children's health information. Much of the information is written for parents.

www.babycenter.com has thousands of articles devoted to pregnancy, childbirth, and children's health. Probably the most comprehensive baby-centered Web site (and we'll admit we're biased toward this site because we both have written for it).

Chapter 5: Breast-feeding: How to Guarantee Success

A few places you can find support:

Make an appointment with a certified lactation consultant. To find a lactation consultant in your area, ask your physician, midwife, or pediatrician for a referral, or call the International Lactation Consultant Association at (919) 787-5181 or visit www.ilca.org.

Talk to other nursing moms. Attend a La Leche League International (LLLI) meeting to meet women who are committed to breast-feeding, and willing to share their experiences—the difficulties and the joys—of breast-feeding. La Leche League is a breast-feeding advocacy and educational organization whose members include both lactation experts and experienced nursing moms. There's a LLLI chapter in virtually every city in the United States and the monthly meetings are free; look in your white pages to find out where your local meeting is held. Call (847) 519-7730 and ask about LLLI's free pamphlets, or call the helpline at (800) 525–3243, or visit www.lalecheleague.org.

Check out online resources. The Nursing Mothers Council (NMC) is one of the most comprehensive breast-feeding Web sites on the internet. An index includes links to dozens of breast-feeding sites, everything from personal Web pages, to the AAP and World Health Organization sites (both include the latest research about the benefits of breast-feeding). Visit: http://www.nursingmothers.org/index.html or call NMC's National Referral Line at (408) 291–8008 to find a local chapter.

Chapter 6: Healing at Home

To find a doula, a specially trained person who can either be a labor coach, or a postpartum support person, contact Doulas of North America by calling (888) 788-DONA or visit www.dona.org.

Chapter 7: Dealing with Mixed Emotions

Postpartum Support International
927 N. Kellogg Avenue
Santa Barbara, California 93111
(805) 967-7636
(805) 967-0608 (fax)
www.postpartum.net

Depression After Delivery
91 East Somerset Street
Raritan, New Jersey 08869
(800) 944-4773 (4PPD)
www.depressionafterdelivery.com

The American Psychological Association
http://helping.apa.org/therapy/depression.html

American Association for Marriage and Family Therapy
For information about how therapy can help with postpartum depression, and for more information about PD, visit http://www.aamft.org/families. Click on "Postpartum Depression."

Chapter 9: Body Wellness

To find hundreds of exercise videos, including some designed just for pregnancy and postpartum, call Collage Video at (800) 433-6769 and request a catalog or visit www.collagevideo.com.

All of the equipment used in The Ultimate Post–C-Section Workout can be purchased at stores such as Wal-Mart and Target. If you'd prefer to shop online, visit www.net2fitness.com or www.gart-sports.com.

For a selection of cute workout maternity and postbaby fitness clothing, plus nursing sports bras, check out Title 9 Sports. Shop online at www.title9sports.com or call (800) 342-4448 to request a catalog. Athleta is another great resource for workout clothing and gear, visit www.athleta.com or call (888) 322-5515.

American Dietetic Association

To find a referral to a registered dietician in your area, visit www.eatright.org or phone (800) 877-1600. Request a dietician who specializes in nutrition during and after pregnancy.

Glossary

abruptio placentae—detachment of a normally situated placenta

American College of Obstetricians and Gynecologists (ACOG)—a private, voluntary, nonprofit membership organization of professionals providing health care for women. The organization has more than 45,000 members and is based in Washington, D.C.

American Academy of Pediatrics (AAP)—an organization of pediatricians with 57,000 members in the United States, Canada, and Latin America. Members include pediatricians, pediatric medical subspecialists, and pediatric surgical specialists

analgesic—a drug that relieves pain

anemia—a condition in which there is a reduction in the number of circulating red blood cells or hemoglobin

anesthetic—an agent that produces partial or complete loss of sensation with or without the loss of consciousness

antibiotics—synthetic or natural substances that inhibit the growth of or destroy microorganisms. Antibiotics are used to treat bacterial infections in humans

birth canal—the canal a fetus goes through during birth, consisting of the cervix, vagina, and vulva

blood thinners—drugs used to prevent clumps of blood from forming or growing in your arteries or veins

breech presentation—a common occurrence in which a fetus' buttocks, rather than his head, are facing downward

cephalopelvic disproportion—a situation in which the size of the fetus' head is too big to fit through the mother's pelvis

cervix—the neck-shaped part of the pelvis

classical incision—a surgical incision used with Cesarean section where the uterus is cut vertically to remove the fetus and placenta

constipation—difficulty passing stools that are very hard and dry

contraception—the devices and medicines used to prevent conceiving a child

deceleration—a decrease in the baby's heart rate

diabetes—a condition marked by insufficient secretion or utilization of insulin; symptoms include frequent urination and excessive amounts of blood and sugar in the urine

diaphragmatic breathing—breathing from the area between the chest and abdomen, known as the diaphragm

dilation—the stretching or enlarging of an organ; when used in relation to pregnancy, the term refers to the cervix dilating

doula—person who assists a woman and her partner with prenatal care, childbirth education, delivery, and postnatal care or postpartum

dystocia—difficult labor

eclampsia—a medical condition marked by convulsive seizures and possibly coma that can develop between the twentieth week of pregnancy and the end of the first week postpartum

ectopic pregnancy—when the fertilized egg implants outside the uterus

epidural anesthesia—an anesthetic that partially or completely numbs the legs and lower abdomen. It's administered by needle into the epidural space that surrounds a fluid-like sac in the spinal column called the dura

episiotomy—an incision of the perineum to help labor along and prevent tearing of the area

estrogen—female sex hormones produced by the ovary or through artificial means

fetal monitoring—the use of electrodes to monitor a fetus's physical condition in response to labor

fetus—a child in utero from the third month to birth

Foley catheter—a tube with a balloon attachment that is passed through the urinary tract to collect urine

forceps—an instrument used during delivery of a fetus to help hold, seize, or extract the baby

fundus—the portion of the uterus that sits above the openings of the fallopian tubes

general anesthesia—an agent that produces a temporary loss of sensation and consciousness

gestational diabetes—a condition that can develop during pregnancy that causes insufficient secretion or utilization of insulin; symptoms include frequent urination and excessive amounts of blood and sugar in the urine

hemorrhage—abnormal internal or external loss of blood from the body

hemorrhoids—dilated veins in the external or internal rectum

hormone—a substance found in an organ or gland that moves through the blood to another area and uses chemical action to increase functional activity or increase secretion of another hormone

hypertension—a condition in which blood pressure is above the normal range

incision—a cut made with a knife, usually for the purpose of surgery

induction—causing the start of labor with the use of oxytocic drugs

intravenous (IV) fluids—water-based solutions administered through the veins

Kegels—exercises designed to strengthen the female perineal muscles

Kerr incision—the side-to-side cut made in the lower uterus during a c-section

lochia—the discharge of blood, mucus, and tissue from the uterus during the six weeks following childbirth

low transverse incision—a type of lateral surgical cut used for a Cesarean section

malpresentation—a situation in which the baby is positioned unusually, i.e., feet first, horizontally, etc.

Maylard incision—a transverse abdominal incision used during a c-section surgery

meconium—an infant's first bowel movement

membranes—a thin, soft, pliable layer of tissue that lines a tube or cavity, covers an organ or structure, or separates one part from another

midwife—a person trained to assist a woman during childbirth. Some also provide prenatal care and help with the baby after birth

misoprostol—a cervix-ripening, synthetic agent used for the induction of labor

morbidity—the incidence of disease within a population

mortality—the rate of the total number of deaths to the total population

neonatalogist—a physician who specializes in the study, care, and treatment of a newborn infant up to six weeks of age

nubain—a potent analgesic used to relieve moderate to severe pain

nurse midwife—a person with a nursing degree and specialized training in midwifery. In the U.S. certified nurse midwives (CNMs) must earn certification from the American College of Nurse Midwives

oxytocin—an agent that stimulates contractions of the uterus

pediatrician—a physician who specializes in the care of children and treatment of their diseases

pelvic floor—a group of three muscles and the connective tissues around the vagina and anus

perineum—the external region between the vulva and anus in a female

Pfannensteil incision—a lateral incision made in the abdomen during a c-section, known widely as the "bikini-cut"

Pitocin—brand name for oxytocin, an agent that stimulates contractions of the uterus

placenta—an oval-shaped, spongelike structure that develops during pregnancy; it attaches to the uterus and provides oxygen and nourishment to the fetus as well as allowing the release of carbon monoxide and waste products from the fetus

placenta accreta—an abnormal adherence of the placenta to the muscle of the uterus

placental abruption—premature separation of the placenta from the uterus

placental insufficiency—a defect of the placenta that causes slowed growth in the fetus

placenta previa—a condition in which the placenta implants in the lower part of the uterus, partially or completely covering the cervix

pre-eclampsia—a condition that occurs during the third trimester of pregnancy marked by high blood pressure, protein in the urine, and swelling of the hands and feet

presentation—the position of the baby during pregnancy

prostaglandin—hormones that ripen the cervix and may cause contractions

spinal anesthesia—an anesthetic used to numb the lower half of the body, given by a needle injected into the dura, a fluid-filled sac that sits in the spinal column

trial of labor—an attempt at labor

ultrasound—a radiology technique that uses high-frequency sound waves to produce images of the fetus in utero

umbilical cord prolapse—a condition in which the umbilical cord falls into the birth canal ahead of the baby's head or other parts of the baby's body

urethra—the tube that transports urine and leads from the bladder to outside the body

urinary incontinence—the inability to retain urine due to loss of spincter control

urinary tract infection—infection of the kidney, ureter, bladder, or urethra

uterine fibroids—a benign tumor residing in the uterus

uterus—a pear-shaped organ located in the lower abdomen

vagina—the muscular canal extending from the cervix to outside the body

··

Selected Bibliography

Introduction

"There are a variety . . ." "Cesarean Section: A Brief History, Part I," U.S. National Library of Medicine, National Institutes of Health, Department of Health and Human Services, 1998. (www.nlm.nih. gov/exhibition/cesarean/cesarean_2.html)

Chapter 1: Why a Cesarean?

"The odds that a baby born . . ." *National Center for Health Statistics, National Vital Statistics Report. Births: Final Data 2002*, Vol. 52, No. 10. December 17, 2003.

"The fact that the technique . . ." James, David, M.A., M.D., F.R.C.O.G., et al., *High Risk Pregnancy: Management Options.* Philadelphia: W.B. Saunders, 1999. Page 1217.

"While the first . . ." "Cesarean Section: A Brief History, Part I." U.S. National Library of Medicine. National Institutes of Health, Department of Health and Human Services. 1998 (www.nlm.nih.gov/exhibition/cesarean/cesarean_2.html)

"For these deliveries . . ." Ibid., Part II.

"By the mid-nineteenth century . . ." Ibid, Part III.

Why a Cesarean Today? Gabbe, Steven G., Niebyl, Jennifer R., et al. *Obstetrics: Normal and Problem Pregnancies, Fourth Edition.* New York: Churchill Livingstone, 2002, pp. 544–46.

"Previous Cesarean . . ." "Evaluation of Cesarean Delivery." Freeman, Roger, M.D., et al. American College of Obstetricians and Gynecologists, 2000, page 21.

"Even though the number of women . . ." *National Center for Health Statistics, National Vital Statistics Report. Births: Final Data 2002*, Vol. 52, No. 10. December 17, 2003.

"Interestingly, one study . . ." Hueston, W.J., et al. "Variations in Cesarean Delivery for Fetal Distress," *Journal of Family Practice*, November 1996, Vol. 43, pp. 461–67.

Table 1: National Center for Health Statistics, *National Vital Statistics Report. Births: Final Data 2002*, Volume 52, No. 10. December 17, 2003. There were 4,021,726 total births in 2002; 1,043,846 babies were delivered via c-section.

"A recent study of breech births . . ." Hannah, Mary E., et al., "Planned ceasarean section versus planned vaginal birth for breech presentation at term: a randomised multicentre trial." *The Lancet*, October 21, 2000 Vol. 356, No. 9239, pp. 1375–83.

"Researchers at the University of Washington . . ." Brown, Zane A., et al. "Effect of serologic status and cesarean delivery on transmission rates of herpes simplex virus from mother to infant." *Journal of the American Medical Association*, January 8, 2003, Vol. 289, No., 2, pp. 203–9.

"Another caveat of the study . . ." ibid.

"In light of the rising rates of c-sections . . ." from "Surgery and Patient Choice: The Ethics of Decision Making," a statement from the American College of Obstetricians and Gynecologists, November 2003.

"A Global Perspective . . ." United Nations Population Fund, "Maternal Mortality Statistics by Region and Country. Estimates developed by the World Health Organization, UNICEF, Save the Children, and the United Nations Population Fund.

"Rates and Implications of Caesarean Sections in Latin America: Ecological Study," *British Medical Journal*, November 27, 1999, pp. 1397–1402.

"Hard Labour? Must be a boy!" Eogan, Maeve A., et al. "Effect of fetal sex on labor and delivery: retrospective review." *British Medical Journal*, Vol. 326, January 18, 2003, page 137.

Chapter 2: The Surgery

"More than four million babies were born in the United States . . ." *National Center for Health Statistics: National Vital Statistics Report*, Vol. 52, No. 10, December 17, 2003.

"In roughly 90 percent of c-section deliveries . . ." Gabbe, Steven G., M.D., Niebyl, Jennifer, R. et. al., *Obstetrics: Normal and Problem Pregnancies Fourth Edition*. New York: Churchill Livingstone, 2002, page 458.

"You may have heard that an epidural . . ." Ibid, page 466.

"One of the more recent studies . . ." *American Journal of Obstetrics and Gynecology*; "Does Epidural Analgesia Prolong Labor and Increase Risk of Cesarean Delivery?" Volume 185, Issue 1, July 2001, pp. 128–134.

"If you do opt to shave . . ." Gabbe, Steven G., M.D., Niebyl, Jennifer R., et, al., *Obstetrics: Normal and Problem Pregnancies Fourth Edition*. New York: Churchill Livingstone, 2002, page 548.

"Your nurse inserts a Foley catheter . . ." *Planning Your Pregnancy and Birth, Third Edition*: The American College of Obstetricians and Gynecologists, page 201.

"She'll place a tiny monitor on your index finger . . ." Ibid, page 201.

"In 90 percent of all Cesarean births . . ." Gabbe, Steven G., M.D., Niebyl, Jennifer R., et. al., *Obstetrics: Normal and Problem Pregnancies Fourth Edition*. New York: Churchill Livingstone, 2002, page 551.

"This type of uterine incision is done in just 10 percent . . ." Ibid, page 551.

"Maternal mortality associated with . . ." *The American College of Obstetricians and Gynecologists, Evaluation of Cesarean Delivery*: "Modes of Delivery: What Are the Risks Associated with Cesarean Delivery?", page 5.

Chapter 3: Healing at the Hospital

"*Thanks to the Newborns' . . .*" U.S. Department of Labor Fact Sheet: Newborns' and Mothers' Health Protection Act.

"Factors that increase your risk . . ." WB Saunders, 2nd Edition, Jan 15, 2000, "The Core Curriculum for Maternal-Newborn Nursing," Mattson, Susan (Ed). Obstetric and Neonatal Nurses Association of Women's Health (AWHONN).

Chapter 4: Your C-Section Baby

"In babies who are born . . ." Faxelius, G. et al. "Catecholamine surge and lung function after delivery," Archives of Disease in Childhood, Volume 58, No. 4, April 1983, pp. 262–66.

"One suggests . . ." Cohen M. and Carson, B. S., "Respiratory morbidity benefit of awaiting onset of labor after elective Cesarean section." *Obstetrics & Gynecology,* Volume 65, No. 6, June 1985, pp. 818–24.

"Another study suggests . . ." Morrison, J. J., et al., "Neonatal respiratory morbidity and mode of delivery at term: influence of timing of elective caesarean section." *British Journal of Obstetrics and Gynaecology,* February 1995, Volume 102, No. 2, pp. 101–6.

"Babies who are born . . ." Levine, E. M., et al., "Mode of delivery and risk of respiratory diseases in newborns." *Obstetrics & Gynecology,* March 2001, Volume 97, No. 3, pp. 439–42.

"Among the things that perhaps . . ." *Nelson Textbook of Pediatrics, 15th edition.* Waldo E. Nelson, senior editor, Richard E. Behrman, Robert M. Kliegman, Ann M. Marvin, editors. Philadelphia: W.B. Saunders, 1996, pp. 434–39.

"Your newborn's first important test." Ibid.

"In fact one study suggested that . . ." Levine, E.M., et al., "Mode of delivery and risk of respiratory diseases in newborns." *Obstetrics & Gynecology,* March 2001, Vol. 97, No. 3, pp. 439–42.

"One condition that can affect . . ." *Nelson Textbook of Pediatrics, 15th edition.* Waldo E. Nelson, senior editor, Richard E. Behrman, Robert M. Kliegman, Ann M. Marvin, editors. Philadelphia: W.B. Saunders, 1996, pp. 434–39.

Table: "Where you live . . ." *National Vital Statistics Report,* Vol. 52, No. 10, December 17, 2003.

Chapter 5: Breast-feeding: How to Guarantee Success

"Although the American Academy of Pediatrics recommends . . ." American Academy of Pediatrics Policy Statement, "Breast-feeding and the Use of Human Milk" (RE9729).

Pediatrics, Vol. 100, No. 6, December 1997, pp. 1035–39.

Healthy People 2010 Objectives for the Nation, U.S. Centers for Disease Control, "Breast-feeding." http://www/cdcgov/breast-feeding/policy-hp2010.htm

"Some of the most recent research . . ." Mortensen, Erik Lykke, et al., "The Association Between Duration of Breast-feeding and Adult Intelligence," *Journal of the American Medical Association*, Vol. 287, No. 18, May 8, 2002, pp. 2365–71.

"You benefit, too . . ." "Breast-feeding: HHS Blueprint for Action on Breast-feeding." Department of Health and Human Services, Office on Women's Health.

"When one study compared 20 infants . . ." Sozmen, M., "Effects of early suckling of cesarean-born babies on lactation," *Biology of the Neonate*. 1992, Vol. 62, No. 1, pp. 67–68.

"One Japanese study . . ." Hirose, M., et al., "Extradural buprenorphine suppresses breast-feeding after caesarean section," *British Journal of Anaesthesia*, Vol. 79, No. 1, February 1998. pp. 120–21.

"A study that looked at the frequency of suckling . . ." Klaus, M.H., "The frequency of sucking: A neglected but essential ingredient of breast-feeding," *Obstetrics and Gynecology Clinics of North America*, Vol. 14, No. 3, September 1987, pp. 623–33.

"Breast-feeding after a Cesarean Birth," La Leche League International, June 1988.

"A Mother's Guide to Pumped Milk," La Leche League International, March 2001.

"Drugs and breast milk, what you need to know," "The transfer of drugs and other chemicals into Human Breast Milk," American Academy of Pediatrics Policy Statement, *Pediatrics*, Volume 108, No. 3, September 2001.

"Can breast-feeding prevent pregnancy?" Townsend, S., "Breast-feeding as a postpartum contraceptive method," *Network*, Vol. 11, No. 3, August 1990, page 16.

Chapter 9. Getting Your Body Back

"Many of them wanted . . ." Moran, C.F., et al., "What do women want to know after childbirth," *Birth*, Vol. 24, 1997, No. 1, pp. 27–34.

"Women who exercise during the postpartum period . . ." Sampelle, C.M., et al., "Physical Activity and Postpartum Well-being," *Journal of Obstetric, Gynecologic and Neonatal Nursing*, Vol. 28, No. 1, January-February 1999, page 41.

"According to the U.S. National Institutes of Health. . . ." "Facts about dietary supplements: iron." Clinical Nutrition Service, Warren Grant Magnuson Clinical Center, National Institutes of Health (NIH), Bethesda, MD, in conjunction with the Office of Dietary Supplements (ODS) in the Office of the Director of NIH.

"If a woman's uterus does rupture . . ." Smith, G. C. et al., "Risk of perinatal death associated with labor after previous cesarean delivery in uncomplicated term pregnancies," *Journal of the American Medical Association*, Vol. 287, No. 20, May 22–29, 2002, pp. 2684–90.

"Want to try a VBAC?" "Evaluation of Cesarean Delivery." Freeman, Roger, M.D., et al., American College of Obstetricians and Gynecologists, 2000.

"One well-publicized study . . ." "Risk of Uterine Rupture during Labor among Women with a Prior Cesarean Delivery," *The New England Journal of Medicine*, Vol. 345, No. 1, July 5, 2001, pp. 3–8.

Chapter 11: Future Pregnancies

"In the obstetrics community . . ." Sachs, Benjamin, Kobelin, Cindy, et al., "The Risks of Lowering the Cesarean-Delivery Rate," Sounding Board, *The New England Journal of Medicine*, Vol. 340, No. 1, January 7, 1999.

"Because there is a small risk . . ." Lydon-Rochelle, Mona, et al., "Risk of Uterine Rupture during Labor among Women with a Prior Cesarean Delivery," *The New England Journal of Medicine*, Vol. 345, No. 1, July 5, 2001, pp. 3–8.

"A previous Cesarean can increase . . ." Hemminki, E., and Merilainen, "Long-term effects of cesarean sections: ectopic pregnancies and placental problems," *American Journal of Obstetrics and Gynecology*, May 1996, Vol. 174, No. 5, pp. 1569–74.

"When considering future pregnancies . . ." Shipp, Thomas D., et al., "Interdelivery Interval and Risk of Symptomatic Uterine Rupture,"

Obstetrics & Gynecology, Volume 97, No. 2, February 2001, pp. 175–177.

"Some physicians believe this . . ." Freeman, Roger, et al., "Evaluation of Cesarean Delivery," American College of Obstetricians and Gynecologists, 2000.

"Refuse cervical ripening . . ." Lydon-Rochelle, Mona, et al., "Risk of Uterine Rupture during Labor among Women with a Prior Cesarean Delivery," *The New England Journal of Medicine*, Vol. 345, No. 1, July 5, 2001, pp. 3–8.

"If a woman's uterus does rupture . . ." Smith, G.C. et al., "Risk of perinatal death associated with labor after previous cesarean delivery in uncomplicated term pregnancies," *Journal of the American Medical Association*, Vol. 287, No. 20, May 22–29, 2002, pp. 2684–90.

"Want to try a VBAC?" "Evaluation of Cesarean Delivery." Freeman, Roger, M.D., et al., American College of Obstetricians and Gynecologists, 2000.

"One well-publicized study . . . " "Risk of Uterine Rupture during Labor among Women with a Prior Cesarean Delivery," *The New England Journal of Medicine*, Vol. 345, No. 1, July 5, 2001, pp. 3–8.

Index